WAA JUN 1 3 2003

D1043651

PRAISE FOR *The Fine Arts*
of Relaxation, Concentration, an

"An excellent primer for waking up. Practice these techniques and your life will change."—Richard Strozzi Heckler, Ph.D., author of *Anatomy of Change*

"By far the best plain-language and practical book on mental training."
—*Mind-Body Wellness*

"What a beautiful book! We need so much in our world to focus on how to *be* instead of how to *do*, and [this book] shows the way."—Larry Dossey, M.D., author of *Healing Words*

"Skillfully weaves together contemporary insights into the value of and need for meditation in our lives with many extremely evocative suggestions for different ways to practice."—Jon Kabat-Zinn, author of *Wherever You Go, There You Are*

"A thoroughly useful, practical guidebook offering a distillation of many years of study and pra

"This is a wond⋯   ⋯m the inside out,' of 'being in⋯   ⋯our inner life and consequent⋯   ⋯ think of no more importan⋯   ⋯ness leader."
—Charles Terry⋯   ⋯dation

158.12 Lev

Levey, Joel.
The fine arts of
relaxation,
concentration &
meditation :

"[The Leveys'] work has great prospects for bringing the inner sciences to a very wide section of people who may not under ordinary circumstances come into contact with the inner technologies of mental development and transformation."—His Holiness the Dalai Lama

"I urge you not only to read this book, but even more, to live with it and see how it softly strikes into your mind, your heart and your ability to put your talents to work."—William C. Miller, author *The Creative Edge*

"The methods included here work wonders. As a satisfied user of so many of them, I affirm that they truly deepen the appreciation of life."—Ram Dass, author of *Still Here*

"A useful guide full of practical strategies for making the personal changes necessary for making lasting and beneficial social and organizational changes."
—Tom Campbell, M.C.P, Executive Assistant to the Washington State Speaker of the House

DISCARDED

PALM BEACH COUNTY
OUTDATED LIBRARY SYSTEM
3650 SUMMIT BLVD.
WEST PALM BEACH, FLORIDA 33406

"Many of the current problems in business and society are the result of limited thinking. Our rapidly evolving, interdependent world requires that we learn to think in a new and integrated way. This book helps open the door."— Michael Lindfield, Internal Organization Development Consultant for Boeing Aerospace, and author of *Dance of Change*

"With clarity, compassion and remarkable insight, the Leveys offer the reader dozens of delightful entrees into the world of meditation. They free meditation from the commonly held notions of rigidity, and set it soaring—fresh and joyful—into the heart and mind of the modern-day spiritual explorer." —Peg Jordan, Author of *The Fitness Instinct*

"There is no question that relaxation and meditation are desperately needed in today's stressful society. The Leveys' book wisely emphasizes the need for relaxation and concentration exercises as skills needed to practice good meditation. Numerous good techniques are presented in this book."—C. Norm Shealy, M.D., Ph.D., Coauthor, *The Creation of Health*, and Founder and Medical Director of Shealy Pain & Health Rehabilitation Institute

"Practical and down-to-earth, this is a remarkable and comprehensive workbook for mastering the stress of life."—*NAPRA ReVIEW*

"In this beautiful book, the Leveys condense two decades of study, experience, and teaching in the art of self mastery. Hopefully everyone who reads this book will make room in their life for the practices and growth program that it illustrates."—Dr. Elmer Green, Coauthor of *Beyond Biofeedback*, Director of the Voluntary Control Program, Menninger Foundation

"The Leveys are making inner quality control technology available to the West." —Bill Veltrop, Founder, International Center for Organization Design

"What we are striving for, whether we know it our not, is to make our life a work of art, so that every move we make is both appropriate and contributes to our increasing satisfaction and mastery. This unique book opens the possibility for doing that. The Leveys provide the most up-to-date guide to living yet base it on techniques that have stood the test of centuries, even millennia." —Michael Ray, Ph.D., Coauthor, *Creativity in Business*, and Professor of Creativity and Innovation and of Marketing, Graduate School of Business, Stanford University

THE FINE ARTS OF RELAXATION, CONCENTRATION, AND MEDITATION

THE FINE ARTS ▼ ▼

OF RELAXATION,

CONCENTRATION,

& MEDITATION

ANCIENT SKILLS FOR MODERN MINDS

Joel & Michelle Levey

 Wisdom Publications • Boston

Wisdom Publications
199 Elm Street
Somerville, Massachusetts 02144
www.wisdompubs.org

© 2003 Joel and Michelle Levey

All rights reserved.

No part of this book may be reproduced in any form or by any means,
electronic or mechanical, including photography, recording, or by any information storage and retrieval system or technologies now known or later developed, without the permission in writing from the publisher.

Library of Congress Cataloging-in-Publication Data
Levey, Joel.
  The fine arts of relaxation, concentration & meditation : ancient
skills for modern minds / Joel & Michelle Levey.
      p. cm.
Includes bibliographical references.
   ISBN 0-86171-349-4 (pbk. : alk. paper)
   1. Success—Psychological aspects. 2. Self—realization. 3.
Relaxation. 4. Attention. 5. Medication. I. Levey, Michelle. II.
Title.
   BF637.S8 L447 2003
   158.1'2—dc21

                                                      2002155615

08 07 06 05 04 03
6   5   4   3   2   1

Cover design by Laura Shaw
Interior design by Gopa & Ted2

Drawing on page 35 by Andrew Campbell

Wisdom Publications' books are printed on acid-free
paper and meet the guidelines for permanence and
durability set by the Council of Library Resources.

Printed in Canada

▼▼ To our many kind teachers
and to the awakening of wisdom
within us all

CONTENTS ▼ ▼ ▼

FOREWORD ▼ ▼ ▼

You are holding in your hands a life raft—a generous, life-saving gift from Joel and Michelle Levey. In our daily lives, we all are forced to navigate turbulent seas. There doesn't seem to be any firm ground in sight, and at any moment in our day, we can be abruptly knocked off course from our plans and our ideals. But as the seas mount in strength and the winds of change become more fierce, there are ways to feel grounded and peaceful. Many of these ways are offered in this book; they are a strong, and very practical life raft.

It's important to realize how our modern techniques of goal-setting and planning—the techniques we learned to employ as we wrestle the world into the shape we wanted—don't work in turbulence. In fact, they do just the opposite of what we might hope: as our plans get tossed by the winds of change, we become more stressed, less effective. We don't know how to navigate in uncertainty and ambiguity.

And yet, this knowledge exists. For millennia, many great teachers and people struggled with their own fears, and they developed practices and ways of being that are absolutely relevant to our present situation.

This is the great gift of this book. It is a gentle and generous offering of practices and perspectives that have helped people find peace for thousands of years. But in receiving this gift, you must offer a gift to yourself: the gift of *time*—time to pause, to reflect, to practice what's offered here. For most of us, time seems to have disappeared. This is the Age of Frenetic Activity. Our lives are over-committed, our children's schedules match our own in craziness, and we feel pressure to be available 24/7. Most of us resent this hyper-activity and, if we ever have time to sit quietly, we wonder about the meaning of these frenetic lives we're leading. Is all this activity leading somewhere worthwhile? At the end of our lives, will we feel satisfied with what we've accomplished? Will we have contributed to the greater good? Are we becoming more effective in our lives and more helpful, or are we just becoming increasingly and senselessly more busy?

Joel and Michelle provide expert guidance in three types of practices that have generally disappeared from our busy lives. We are guided from dynamic relaxation, to concentration, to meditation. My own experience with these practices is that once I experienced relaxation, I was eager to go to a deeper, quieter place. These exercises provide so much benefit that you only need to try one or two, and then your whole being will yearn for the next level of peace. When I do any one of these practices, I'm startled to realize what I've been letting pass me by—silence, breathing, reflection, calmness, centeredness.

We are each responsible for cultivating peace; no one will do it for us. The demands of the world—of work and family—constantly call me away from peace. It doesn't take much to pull me off center—it can be the first phone call of the morning, an angry driver on my way to work, a news report, a crying child. But having tasted peace, I now *notice* what it feels like to be pulled off balance. I notice the way it feels to be anxious, resentful, angry, or fearful. I feel the contrast between these emotions and inner peace; I hear it in my voice, feel it in my energy, see it in my thoughts. Having learned how to cultivate peace, I know now that I can consciously choose for peace, in any situation, at any time. But not if I haven't taken time to do some of the practices that lead me into peace.

Of course I'm too busy, and of course the time I spend on cultivating my peace varies widely with the circumstances of my life. But now, when I find myself slipping into impatience, or fear, or anger, I know it's time to pay attention to my practice, to the practices introduced in this book. I know another way of being in my life is possible, if I'm willing to exercise discipline and carve out the time for practice.

I hope you will give yourself the gift of time, experiment with a few of these practices, and discover how much more capable you become to deal with life once you know what inner peace feels like. This world certainly needs more peaceful people. May you contribute to that and so benefit many.

Margaret J. Wheatley

AWAKENING OUR FULL POTENTIAL ▼ ▼ ▼

A human being is part of the whole called by us "universe," a part limited in time and space. We experience ourselves, our thoughts and feelings as something separate from the rest. A kind of optical delusion of consciousness. This delusion is a kind of prison for us, restricting us to our personal desires and to affection for a few persons nearest to us. Our task must be to free ourselves from the prison by widening our circle of compassion to embrace all living creatures and the whole of nature in its beauty.... We shall require a substantially new manner of thinking if mankind is to survive.

Albert Einstein

In each of our lives there have been times when we have experienced a deeper sense of connectedness, wholeness, and belonging than we ordinarily find. Most likely those extraordinary moments of deeper wisdom, love, and aliveness came unexpectedly. Pause for a moment to recall those special moments when you were most fully and joyfully alive...when you felt the exhilaration of performing at your best...when you allowed your heart to open to tenderly love and be loved...when you were in the *flow* and felt in perfect harmony with the world in which you live. Recall those quintessential moments in your life and work that stand out and sparkle...those times when you really helped someone or when you really allowed someone to care for you. If we examine the qualities of our minds during these special times we will probably find that our attention was wholly focused on what was happening and that our mind and body were operating as one. Remembering and appreciating such special moments in our lives serves to remind us of what is possible.

But why are these moments so rare? Generally speaking, our attention is quite scattered—we are lost in our thoughts and only superficially in touch with the reality and intensity of our inner and outer experiences. Our minds are so infrequently calm and clear enough to discern the play of inspiration and revelation that are a natural, though very subtle, part of our lives. How many valuable insights and breakthrough ideas have we missed because the noise level in our mindbody was simply too high to discern these sublime whispers that are an ongoing function of our human life?

Similarly, we all too often wait until the whispers of tension in our bodies, our relationships, and our world become heart-wrenching screams of pain before we wake up and fully acknowledge them or attempt to restore harmony and balance. How many moments of struggle, pain, and grief—how many billions of dollars in wasted time, energy, and resources—would be saved if we, as individuals and organizations, devoted more attention to refining and developing our capabilities for inner awareness and enhanced mental development? Though our bodies are really not very different from those of our ancestors, we live in a dramatically different and infinitely more complex and demanding world. In a single day we may be challenged to respond to more information and make more decisions than one of our ancestors faced in years. Given the accelerating rate of change and uncertainty, the immensity of personal and global crises, and the staggering variety of choices and decisions that are a part of our daily life, is it any wonder that we often feel overwhelmed and frustrated?

With so may people needlessly suffering and dying from preventable stress-related diseases, millions of people are searching for wiser, kinder, and less self-destructive ways of living in today's world. When we consider the enormous costs incurred by our bodies, our minds, our relationships, and our environment, it is no surprise that so many people are seeking to increase their resilience, deepen their wisdom, and get in touch with life-affirming forces. It is no shock that skills in relaxation, concentration, and meditation are being more widely embraced as vital for enhancing the quality of our health, work, relationships, and peace of mind.

DEVELOPING THE MIND

▼▼ The greatest revolution in our generation is the discovery that human beings by changing the inner attitudes of their minds can change the outer aspects of their lives.

William James

While many people regard the state of their mind as an unalterable condition, the world's ancient contemplative traditions and modern cognitive sciences have demonstrated that through proper training and discipline, we can radically enhance the quality of our attention, emotional intelligence, creativity, and intuitive intelligence. The development of these and other mental capabilities offers an advantage for increasing our resilience, health, vitality, effectiveness, and well-being in complex times like these.

Through training, individuals are capable not only of improving their health, but of enhancing creativity and creative problem-solving, extending the length and quality of their lives, awakening greater empathy and compassion, and expanding the scope of their contribution to the world. The multiple and complex dilemmas of modern life represent a need, and the inner sciences of mindbody development offer a variety of profoundly practical and compassionate solutions. Once learned, these inner skills are generative, self-reinforcing, inexpensive, portable, reliable, easily valuable, diffusible, and value-adding in virtually every personal and professional situation.

▼▼ We don't understand the operations of our minds and hence we don't operate them very well.

Charles Tart

To accomplish the inner work we must rely upon the primary tool of our own bodymind. This is a universal tool of infinite potential. With it we create and guide the use of all other tools. Yet, growing up, in school or on the job, few of us have learned even the most basic skills to ensure its optimal performance, maintenance, and fine-tuning.

Consider, did our parents, teachers, health care providers, or clergy ever teach you techniques to let go of stress and tension, to harness and focus the power of your mind, or to gain deep insight through meditation? Did they themselves practice or even appreciate the value of these skills? Most likely not. Lacking such fundamental human training, we in modern times, have much to learn from the traditional inner sciences of mind.

▼▼ In this century, human knowledge is extremely expanded and developed but this is mainly knowledge of the external world.... We spend a large amount of the best human brain power looking outside—too much, and it seems we do not spend adequate effort to look within, to think inwardly.... Perhaps now that the Western sciences have reached down into the atom and out into the cosmos finally to realize the extreme vulnerability of all life and value, it is becoming credible, even obvious, that the Inner Science is of supreme importance. Certainly physics designed the bombs, biology the germ warfare, chemistry the nerve gas and so on, but it will be the unhealthy emotions of individuals that will trigger these horrors. These emotions can only be controlled, reshaped, and rechanneled, by technologies developed from successful Inner Science.

The Dalai Lama

TOOLS FOR INNER WORK

For simplicity of presentation in this book, we have organized the sequence of training into three progressively more encompassing domains: dynamic relaxation, concentration, and meditation.

By mastering the art of *dynamic relaxation* we learn to recognize and reduce unproductive tensions, anxieties, and struggles in our inner world and in our outer lives. By learning to free ourselves from the burden of accumulated tensions and inner conflicts, we are better equipped to think more clearly, reduce distress, increase our efficiency and productivity, and generally enhance our well-being.

Mastering the inner art of *concentration* we learn to harness and direct the power of the mind. Transforming the chaotic agitation of our ordinary thinking into a focused beam of awareness, we are able to direct our attention wholeheartedly and productively toward whatever we do. Free from agitation and dullness, our mind grows more peaceful and more powerful. Concentration builds a coherence of mind like a laser beam of attention capable of penetrating the profound subtleties of our life and the world in which we live.

A successful practice of the powerful methods of *meditation* will be greatly enhanced by having learned to quiet the noise in the body through relaxation and to build power and peace of mind through concentration. Approached in this way, meditation techniques enable us to awaken the insight necessary to consciously recognize and transform the harmful or unproductive patterns of our lives, and to consciously strengthen the mind's potential for wisdom, compassion, and creativity. And as this happens, our appreciation for the true nature and potential of ourselves and others grows; inner and outer conflicts diminish; and we become more joyful and more empowered in helping others and the world.

Finally, this book contains a fourth section that offers some additional perspectives and strategies for integrating the fine arts of relaxation, concentration, and meditation into your daily life, work, and relationships.

RELAXATION, PEAK PERFORMANCE, AND BEYOND

This book is a mental-fitness manual for everyone interested in learning methods to enhance their health and performance, master stress, and deepen their appreciation of life. This is also a handbook for those who wish to understand and master these skills in order to teach them to others or to equip themselves to make a greater contribution to the world. Whatever your motivation, you will find that the ideas and techniques in this collection have been presented with an emphasis on their practical applications in our busy lives, while preserving a sense of the depth and sacredness associated with these traditional inner arts. We suggest that you explore these ideas with your intellect, contemplate their meaning and value in your heart, and test and confirm their profound practicality in the laboratory of your daily life and the playing fields of your work and relationships.

If you are primarily interested in physical relaxation or in learning to stay centered, calm, and focused amid chaos, you will find many of these techniques highly effective. If exploring the nature and potential of your mindbody is important to you, these methods will help ripen your understanding. If improving your mental and physical performance, or building healthier and more harmonious relationships, is of significance to you, there are many strategies that will help you in these arenas as well. And if you approach this inquiry with a heartfelt sense of devotion, a sincere yearning to deepen your spiritual insight and empower yourself to be of greater service to others, many of these methods will serve as a vehicle of transformation, opening doors to new dimensions of wisdom, love, and inner strength.

FIELD TESTED

This book contains a distillation of over a hundred methods that we have found personally and professionally effective in our work with thousands of people over the past thirty years. During that time we have had the rare opportunity to train closely with many respected masters and researchers of the inner arts and sciences. From these remarkable men and women we have learned thousands of effective techniques for developing the full potential of the human mindbody. In many cases these methods have been practiced, cherished, and preserved by generations of people with inspiring results for millennia.

The contemporary renaissance of interest in matters of mental health and fitness, spirit, and consciousness has brought these methods of relaxation, concentration, and meditation out of isolated caves, remote monasteries, and foreign cultures and into the research institutions and mainstream of our modern lives. They have been scientifically studied and demonstrated to be effective at enhancing health and optimizing mental and physical performance. They are also effective antidotes to the epidemic of stress-related diseases, anxiety, hostility, dysfunctional behavior, and existential yearnings that plague so many in our complex and rapidly changing world.

For more than three decades we have relied upon these inner arts and disciplines as primary tools in our work. We've worked in many capacities: as mental fitness coaches for athletes and corporate peak performers; researchers investigating the nature of human consciousness; psychophysical therapists directing clinical programs in numerous medical centers, faculty members in graduate programs in medicine, psychology of consciousness, holistic health, leadership and organization design; counselors for people facing terminal illness or grieving the loss of a loved one; teachers of the contemplative arts and sciences; and as guides to many people around the globe seeking to increase their vitality and resilience. It has always been our goal to help people live and work in a more integrated, authentic, and deeply spirited way, thereby making a greater contribution to their world.

HOW TO GET THE MOST
FROM THIS BOOK ▼ ▼ ▼

The challenges of millennia and the inspiration of the human spirit have given rise to thousands of techniques of relaxation, concentration, and meditation. Over the past twenty years we have learned, practiced, and taught others many of these methods. In the pages that follow you will find the distillation of those methods that we have found most widely effective.

We suggest that you consider this book as an investment portfolio offering you a wide range of options. Your return will depend largely upon the sincerity and continuity of your investment of attention and aspiration. Though these methods are priceless you must make a personal investment in them in order call forth the power of which these words are merely shadows. The greater your personal investment in taking these principles and techniques to heart, the greater will be your return and the more you will have to offer to the world.

There are three steps in mastering these techniques. Reading or hearing about them is the first step. Contemplating and thinking about their meaning, value, and application in your daily life is the second step. Taking the meaning and value to heart and directly applying this to your life is the third step. All of these steps are important in discovering the power and profundity of each technique. Though benefits may be immediately apparent, the real fruits of these methods will only emerge gradually as you cultivate them with sustained effort. As your practice deepens, the fruits will grow sweeter, and your appreciation of life will grow.

How long will it take to master a technique? How long would it take you to learn to master the flute or a foreign language? The key to all learning is commitment and discipline. While books, tapes, and teachers are invaluable, ultimately it is your own diligence that will assure your success. Have faith in your abilities to use these techniques. Let the difficulties and uncertainties in your life—and the beauty—provide a continual reminder of the vital importance of practicing these skills.

This book is arranged in five sections: *Relaxation, Concentration, Meditation, Wisdom in Daily Life,* and *Meditation in the World of Work.* Each of the first three sections has an introduction to the ideas and methods, a description of the guidelines for using these methods, and then the methods themselves.

We suggest that you first read the introduction and guidelines for each section. As you read, note those ideas and exercises that seem to speak most directly to you. Once you have identified them, begin to put them into practice by reading them slowly and thoughtfully. Proceed step by step to get the feeling behind the words. You may find it helpful to have a friend read the exercise to you, or to record it in your own voice to replay it at your leisure. Or you may feel inspired to change our terminology to better suit your own style or beliefs. As your familiarity with a technique grows, you will learn to progress through its various stages without needing to read or listen to the instructions. Though at first you may mentally talk yourself through an exercise, gradually cultivate the skill to move through the method as a progression of silent shifts in awareness, a series of mental images or feelings rather than mere words and concepts.

The following chart will help you to identify the techniques in this book that will speak most directly to your needs and interests.

If you are interested in...	*experiment with techniques on these pages*
Flow state, peak performance, and achieving breakthrough	29, 55, 68, 101, 113, 129, 131, 134, 151, 171, 173, 180, 182, 222
Enhancing creativity, innovative thinking, and intuition	29, 41, 55, 64, 98, 101, 104, 108, 111, 122, 124, 127, 129, 136, 138, 144, 154, 168, 173, 180, 190, 193, 212
Self-empowerment	27, 35, 64, 73, 82, 96, 104, 108, 111, 113, 117, 119, 122, 124, 134, 147, 155, 157, 164, 171, 203, 208, 223, 230

PART ONE
▼ ▼ ▼ RELAXATION

Do everything with a mind that lets go.
Do not expect any praise or reward.
If you let go a little, you will have a little peace.
If you let go a lot, you will have a lot of peace.
If you let go completely, you will know complete peace and freedom.
Your struggles with the world will have come to an end.

Ajahn Chah

DYNAMIC RELAXATION ▼ ▼ ▼

The relaxation described in the pages that follow is not a passive, limp, or ineffectual state, but one characterized by a dynamic, ever-adapting balance between a calm, clear, relaxed quality of presence and an alert readiness. This state of dynamic relaxation is finely tuned and responsive to the ever-changing circumstances and conditions of daily life. With practice you will learn to immediately feel when you are holding more tension than you need to perform at your best. By learning to release that extra tension, your brain and muscles will be vitalized with oxygen and nutrients, you will be able to think more clearly and make better decisions, and your ability to act will be enhanced.

Relaxation skills are the foundation for practicing concentration and meditation. You probably know from experience how difficult it is to harness and focus the power of your mind when your body is filled with tension and your mind clouded by fatigue and anxiety.

Once you begin to understand and practice the skills described here, the tensions and distress of your life can be met as opportunities to apply and refine your growing skills in relaxation. This requires the conscious cultivation of:

1. Self-awareness: the ability to know what you are experiencing—sensing, feeling, thinking, etc.—at any moment
2. Care and kindness: the authentic and heartfelt concern that deliberately chooses the paths that lead to greater harmony in your mental, physical, and personal relationships with the world
3. A joyful appreciation of the process: an attitude of gratitude and openness to learning and growing from life's unceasing challenges, a joyful

dedication to living life as a game to be mastered in the arenas of your own mindbody, and in your work and relationships

4. Commitment and courage: the willingness to do whatever it takes to continue to realize and nurture your own extraordinary potentials and help others do the same

Relaxation skills build the foundation for your practice of concentration and meditation. This is a dynamic process, leaving us at times immobilized by distress, at times simply coping with our tensions and anxieties, and at times energized, calm, and confident, having all the information and ability we need to master the stressful demands that life's changing conditions inevitably bring. Having learned to master stress, and to live more and more in the state of flow, we catch the upward spiral of continuous personal development. Breakthroughs to extraordinary levels of health, insight, and performance become more the norm than the exception.

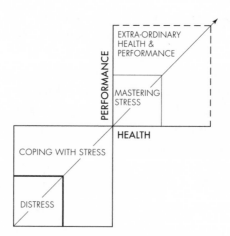

Though stress and tension will always be a part of your life, when you know how to relax, there is no need to get tense about being tense, or feel anxious about feeling anxious. Stress will energize rather than destroy you. Change and challenge will provide every opportunity for growth, creative expression, and extraordinary levels of health, performance, and insight.

As you learn to reduce the noise in your system, physical vitality, mental clarity, calm, centered strength, and emotional well-being that are fundamental to the human spirit will naturally and effortlessly arise.

With this in mind, let's look at the guidelines and methods of practicing the fine arts of relaxation.

▼▼ Remember...

Relaxation is not something that you do.

It is a natural response that you allow to happen.

Relaxation is what is left when you stop creating tension.

GUIDELINES FOR
DEVELOPING RELAXATION SKILLS ▼ ▼ ▼

1. MOTIVATION

When you start to practice relaxation or mental development skills it is important to understand why you are doing it and to generate a positive motivation toward this learning process. Actively choose to practice relaxation. Remember that it is not what you do but how and why you do it that matters.

2. REGULAR PRACTICE

Make these relaxation tools work for you. Regular, consistent practice is essential if you want to gain maximum benefit from these skills. Remember that when you learn to, say, ride a bicycle, develop marksmanship, or any other physical skill, you are using muscles you have never used before. So too when you learn how to relax: You will be stretching mental muscles that you may have never been aware of before.

Many people recommend that you practice twenty minutes in the morning and twenty minutes in the evening—and this ideal would be excellent. But more important is to consciously integrate these techniques into your daily activities. While standing in line, waiting on the phone, or sitting at a stop light, pause for a few moments to breathe away your tensions and bring calm and clarity to your mind. The more frequently you use these strategies, the more dependable they will be for you. Continuity of practice over time will, in the long run, be more important than duration of any one practice session.

3. A QUIET ENVIRONMENT

It is better at first to practice in quiet, comfortable surroundings. This will help you to zero in on the physical and mental qualities you are learning to develop.

Once you have become familiar with your internal controls, and how to access your target state of relaxation, you will be able to carry your practice over into more stressful environments. In fact, the world will continually provide you with opportunities to test and refine your skills in the face of challenge and the unexpected. Having mastered these skills, it is possible that at some critical moment, when it really counts, you will have the energy, balance, and clarity to touch somebody's life in a meaningful way—and this, of course, includes your own!

4. FOCUSING THE MIND

At the beginning of each session, it is helpful to employ a concentration technique to quiet, calm, and focus your mind. A simple method is to be mindful of the natural flow of your breathing as you inhale and exhale with full awareness. You might also experiment with the many excellent concentration techniques presented in Part Two: Concentration.

5. EFFORTLESSNESS AND VOLUNTARY SURRENDER

This state is characterized by an alert, receptive, and calm intensity of awareness. Initially, the challenge is to learn to develop a fine balance between an open, calm attentiveness and the more tightly focused mind that tries to change something or make something happen. This balance is learned through practice and attention to the feedback you receive from your attempts to relax your body and mind.

For best results, *allow relaxation to happen.* The harder you try, the tenser you will become. Release your tensions as you exhale. Relax into the gentle pull of gravity. Let your eyes be soft. In an easy, natural and effortless manner, just let go of the mindbody tensions that you no longer need.

Allow your internal RPMs to slow down, and find your natural rhythm.

If you are the type of person who has always been busy *doing* rather than *being*, this approach may at first be alien to you. With practice, however, you will discover a totally new type of inner strength and power when you are deeply relaxed. Don't worry about losing control. Whenever you need to apply effort or push harder you will be rested enough to do so. You are simply learning to have the choice of two operating modes rather than the compulsive limitation of one inefficient habit. Without this option you may struggle for the rest of your life to keep control rather than simply settling into the power of life naturally and effortlessly.

6. PROPER POSTURE

For best results, a comfortable upright position is recommended for practicing these relaxation techniques. It is important that your spine be straight. Lying down is discouraged if you have a tendency to fall asleep. With practice, you will find that you can tune in to an optimal balance between relaxation and activation while walking, talking, driving, or engaging in any activity.

7. EXTERNAL GUIDANCE, INTERNAL GUIDANCE

Initially, the external guidance of another person or a taped guided relaxation is useful as it is easier to just let go into the experience. As you become familiar with the stages of relaxation and the variety of mental and physical indicators, you will be able to enter these states at will and under your own guidance. The balance that you develop is similar to simultaneously driving a car and being free to enjoy the view, or playing music and being totally entranced by it at the same time.

For most of us, this is an unfamiliar state of awareness. With practice, however, you will expand your mental and physical awareness to allow you to easily guide your own relaxation sessions.

8. TIMING

Once you have become familiar with the relaxation techniques by practicing morning and evening, you will be able to apply them when you need to throughout the day as an antidote to stressful situations. You may wonder, however, just when the best time would be to actually apply them. Generally speaking, it is best to practice *before* you are mentally or physically exhausted. And try to avoid practicing on a full stomach or when you are extremely hungry.

If you wait until you just can't take any more, odds are your mind will be so agitated that it will be almost impossible to concentrate. And if you wait until you are exhausted or full from eating, you will probably fall asleep. As soon as the boat starts to take on water—use the bilge pump! Don't wait until you feel swamped or out of control before you use these techniques to dissipate stress.

Remember that your body-mind is your primary instrument. Monitor it carefully throughout the day. Consciously relax or fine-tune frequently.

If you are having difficulty settling down and tuning in, try scheduling your relaxation sessions immediately after periods of exercise or heightened arousal. At these times there is a tangible mental and physical release, a natural time of letting go. Just ride the wave of this shift from sympathetic-nervous-system activation to the parasympathetic relaxation response. At this time investigate and recognize the stages, feelings, and indicators of relaxation while they are most apparent.

9. OVERCOMING DIFFICULTIES

There are two main obstacles that you will inevitably encounter in your practice—distraction and drowsiness.

Distraction can be of two types: external, such as noise, heat, cold; and internal, such as physical sensations, pain, and mental wandering. The best strategy in both cases is to include the distraction in your awareness while minimizing your resistance to or identification with the distracting event. Just let it be, and keep your attention on what you are doing. Even if your mind wanders a thousand times, gently bring it back. Do not engage in mental commentary on the process—just do it. Gradually, the agitated, wandering mind will be tamed and you will be able to stay focused on the task at hand.

As for *drowsiness* or mental dullness, it would be useful to check your posture to make sure you are sitting upright. You could take a few deep breaths, or even splash your face with cold water before continuing your practice.

You might find it helpful to contemplate the preciousness of your life and the unpredictability of your death, and to muster a firm resolve to make the most of each moment.

Don't allow your wandering, compulsive mind to control your life, and likewise, don't wait to wake up on your deathbed realizing that you have slept through most of your life. *Take charge! Be patient!*

10. CHOOSING A TECHNIQUE

As we begin our practice of these skills, our challenge is to recognize and to master our stress response. Dr. Alice Domar, M.D., explains, "The best antidote to stress—besides altering your life so it's less stressful—is learning to manage it through mind-body methods such as meditation, mindfulness, guided imagery, and deep breathing. Recent Harvard studies have found that these techniques can successfully treat a host of…health problems." Since each of us has a unique style of responding to the stressors of our daily life, different techniques geared to optimize psychophysical states will be effective for different individuals.

For example, if your symptoms of stress include neuromuscular signs, such as muscle aches and pain, tension headaches, backaches, spasms or tics, fatigue, then the methods of modified progressive relaxation, autogenic imagery, the flow sequence, mental massage, and numerous other methods may be quite effective.

If your symptoms of distress are primarily cognitive, such as anxiety, worry, intrusive or repetitive thoughts, then the concentration techniques and the meditations for listening, walking, investigating the mind and thought may be very helpful.

If your symptoms include autonomic-nervous-system symptoms or disease, including hypertension, migraines, gastrointestinal distress, poor circulation, excessive sweating, eating disorders, you might benefit from consistent practice of autogenic imagery, the hollow body meditation, and the practices of giving and taking, loving-kindness, and forgiveness.

If you are prone to negative and unsettling emotions, such as anger, impatience, guilt, obsessive desire, then the concentration techniques may offer temporary relief while the meditations on the mind, thoughts, forgiveness, loving-kindness, compassion, and the practice of giving and taking, may help to uproot the deeper causes of your emotional distress.

Individuals suffering from chronic pain may find some relief from the practice of relaxation techniques in general followed by the use of mental massage, hollow body, and the strategies for transforming pain.

If you feel that you have mastered your response to life's myriad stressors and that your wish is to tap your latent potentials, virtually every method described in this book holds the potential to open new horizons of understanding, performance, and human kindness.

11. RELEASE PHENOMENA

As you begin to relax, it is quite common to experience what are called *release phenomena*. Some examples of these are jerking or quivering of the body as when one falls asleep, gurgling of the stomach, tingling feelings or numbness, perspiration, memories or feelings or perceptual changes spontaneously arising. Remember that it is natural to become aware of certain experiences when we are relaxed that we wouldn't normally notice during times of activity. For example, you may be injured while playing a game but because of the excitement you do not notice the pain until later when you have slowed down.

Release phenomena are common indicators that your practice of relaxation or meditation techniques is becoming effective in dissolving your mental, emotional, and physical tension. The best way to deal with these experiences as they occur is to regard them without judgment—you may find them either disturbing or quite pleasant. Simply allow them to arise, flow freely, and dissolve without distracting your attention.

Most of us are more familiar with the signs of stress than with the indicators of relaxation. With practice, you will become aware of the subtle physical, emotional, and mental states associated with progressively deeper levels of relaxation and meditation. Eventually, your reservoirs of stress will be drained and your circuits cleared, allowing you to handle the challenges of daily life more effectively and with greater patience and understanding. When you are on the right track, a sigh, a tingling, a sense of deep warmth will become a familiar signpost on your daily stroll through your inner landscape.

12. RIGHT RELATIONSHIP

The success of your relaxation and meditation program is directly related to your discipline in your relationship to the world. Plagued as we usually are by anger, fear, jealousy, guilt, or worry, it is extremely difficult to develop the concentration and understanding necessary to master our minds. The conflicts of our daily lives will become painfully clear to us the moment we focus our attention in our practice. Ignoring these conflicts doesn't make them go away. Instead, we are faced with the challenge of truly mastering our lives rather than being a slave to our mental distortions and emotional confusions.

As you exercise more discipline in your relationship to the world, your ability to concentrate and focus the mind will grow. With this enhanced mental clarity and stability, new understanding and insight will reveal better approaches to living. In this way, inner and outer discipline reinforce each other.

13. ALTERATIONS IN CONSCIOUSNESS

▼▼ The man who comes back through the door in the wall will never be quite the same as that man who went out. He will be wiser, but less cocksure, happier but less self-satisfied, humbler in acknowledging his ignorance, yet better equipped to understand the relationship of words to things, of systematic reasoning to the unfathomable Mystery which it tries forever vainly to comprehend.

Aldous Huxley

Since childhood we have learned to selectively attend to certain aspects of reality and to ignore others. Yet at times in each of our lives the trance of the cultural hypnosis that Einstein called the "optical delusion of consciousness" has lifted and we have glimpsed for a timeless moment a deeper understanding of ourselves and our world. We behold what we value: The Eskimos describe dozens of kinds of snow, the Tibetans have catalogued 121 different states of consciousness, and some cultures regard their dream worlds as real as their ordinary waking experiences.

Many of the techniques in this book are actually methods for deconditioning, ways of relaxing the limitations of our view of who we are, how we can perform, and what is happening in the world around us. All the techniques here can be included in two categories. Concentrative techniques help us focus our attention, and receptive techniques help us scan the full spectrum of the world in a wide-open way. In fact, the complete picture is being broadcast to us on many tracks simultaneously, but for most of our life we have been monitoring only one of these tracks at a time.

During moments of peak performance, relaxation, dreams, intuition, physical exercise, meditation, sexual experience, or prayer, the spectrum of our awareness may naturally expand to encompass new and deeper ways of experiencing and knowing.

Psychologist William James sums up the challenge of integrating a full spectrum of awareness into our daily lives this way:

▼▼ Our normal waking consciousness, rational consciousness as we call it, is but one special type of consciousness, whilst all about it parted by the flimsiest of screens, there lie potential forms of consciousness entirely different. We may go through life without suspecting their existence: but apply the requisite stimuli and at a touch they are there in all their completeness, definite types of mentality, which probably somewhere have their field of adaptation. No account of the universe in its totality can be final, which leaves other forms of consciousness quite disregarded. How to regard them is the question—for they are so discontinuous with ordinary consciousness. Yet they may determine attitudes though they cannot furnish formulas and open a region though they fail to give a map. At any rate, they forbid a premature closing of our accounts of reality.

14. DYNAMIC ACTION

Relaxation and meditation sessions are times to focus your mind, fine-tune your energies and prepare for dynamic and effective action. It is the time that allows you to be out on the spinning rim of life and still feel the stillness, power, and calm at the center of your being.

As you end a session, consciously carry that energy into action. Throughout the day, frequently scan your circuits, fine-tune as necessary, and embody the awareness and effectiveness of the skills you have been working so hard to master.

15. THE FIVE POWERS

We can identify five mental powers that are essential for developing mental fitness: (1) confidence/trust, (2) energy, (3) concentration, (4) mindfulness/attention, and (5) insight/understanding. These five powers can be effective antidotes to certain common hindrances: (1) doubt/fear, (2) lethargy/procrastination, (3) distraction/ agitation, (4) forgetfulness and (5) confusion.

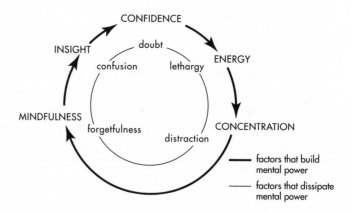

Would you ever begin anything if you lacked even the basic confidence in your ability to accomplish it or at least to learn from the experience? A sense of confidence is essential if your practice of the fine arts of relaxation, concentration, and meditation is to have results. The sense of trust and confidence counteracts your doubts and helps you transform every experience gained during your practice into grist for the mill of your insight and growth.

Hope and fear, pain and ecstasy, every moment of change and flow reveals to you the nature of your mind and body. This understanding can set you free from old emergency reactions and compulsive behavior.

▼▼ Understanding of process enables a person to gain control of that process or to gain freedom from being controlled by it. Thus, analytic understanding of the atomic components of blind rage—what triggers it, how it directs itself, how it mobilizes mental, verbal and physical energies and so on enables an habitually angry person to begin to control his or her temper, perhaps finally to become free of its control.

The Dalai Lama

Though you may have little control over the specific contents of your thoughts, images, and feelings, you will discover that you have the power to alter the process through which you relate to the contents of your mind.

Beginning your practice with a joyful mind and a sense of confidence will help you to tap the second power, energy. It will help you overcome the hindrance of lethargy or procrastination and will move you along on the spiral of growth.

Having generated the powers of confidence and energy, they must be blended with the powers of concentration and mindfulness. Concentration provides a focus and the clarity to direct the energy of your intention. Mindfulness provides the continuity of attention that enables you to be fully present with whatever you are doing. Concentration counteracts distraction and dullness, and mindfulness is the antidote to forgetting what you are doing.

As we begin our practice of these relaxation skills, our challenge is to recognize and to master our unique pattern of stress response. For some people this will mean learning to lower their blood pressure and calm their racing heart when faced with a stressful situation. For others, relaxation may be more about learning to unclench their tight muscles in order to be more comfortable, present, and at ease in challenging situations. Understanding that your initial beliefs, calculations, or intuitions were valid, or having gained insight into how they must be modified, the power of your self-confidence will naturally grow. Your insight will overpower the immobilizing obstacles of your doubt and fear. This power of confidence based on previous success and understanding can then serve to propel you on through a growth curve of heightened energy, concentration, mindfulness, and wisdom.

Having maintained your initial intention through the powers of confidence, energy, concentration, and mindfulness, the fifth power of insight will naturally and effortlessly ripen. The disciplined mind will have the integrity to reach deep and sometimes profound insights regarding this remarkable process called yourself.

16. THE POWER OF THE INNER SMILE

Perhaps the most important guideline to remember is to bring a tender, inner smile to your practice of these techniques. This smile will protect you from trying too hard to relax, or from worrying that you may not be doing it right. Appreciate your success, and learn from the difficulties that you may encounter. If at the end of a relaxation session you are 20 or 30 percent more relaxed, celebrate your success rather than feeling frustrated because some tension still remains.

The compendium of relaxation techniques described in this book is intended to familiarize you with a variety of skills and strategies. Read through and choose those that seem to speak most directly to your own needs and interests. Again, feel free to adapt any words or images to your own style. With practice you will become familiar with the unique characteristics and indicators of each of these techniques and you will be able to recommend or teach appropriate ones to others.

Bring a joyful sincerity to your practice of these skills.

Remember how short and precious your life really is.

1 LETTING GO OF TENSION ▼ ▼ ▼

This technique will help you recognize the various levels of tension that you experience throughout the day and will help you learn how to relax deeply.

First, tense your whole body as tightly as possible. Clench your fists, flex your feet and toes. Make a face—squeeze tightly but not so tightly that you hurt yourself. Squeeze…tense…and hold for a few moments. Notice what it feels like to be this tense. Hold…and now relax, relax completely…allow your breath to fill you naturally, and as you exhale, let go completely. Let go into gravity. Release any tensions that you don't need. Allow the waves of breath to ebb and flow.

Now, once again, tense your whole body, but this time tense only half as much as before. Tense…hold…feel what it is like to hold this level of tension. Hold…and let go. As you breathe, let go completely of any tensions in your mind and body. Allow each breath to carry away all your tension. Now, feel what it is like to have released and let go of tension.

Once again, tense your whole body, but again only half as much as the last time. Tense…hold…feel how it is to have this level of tension in your body. Feel the bracing, squeezing, holding. Recognize that frequently throughout the day you are probably as tense as this without knowing it. Now, exhale…let go completely. Allow the waves of breath to wash away the tension. Let go into gravity. Feel your body opening to the flow of life. Feel your vitality and a deep, pervasive warmth within you.

Again, tense your body, and again, only half as much as the time before. Scan your body and feel the subtle ways in which tension pervades it. Hold…feel it…and let go completely. Gently relax into the flow of your breath. Allow your body and mind to find their perfect harmony.

Now, tense only your mind. Clench your attention around a thought or anxiety. Hold…feel the subtle pain in your heart closing around fear, anger, doubt, guilt. Generate a wish to be free from this pain and tension. Now breathe…open…release. Allow your mind and heart to open to the flow of thoughts, images, and feelings within the sphere of your experience. Rest in this openness. Watch as fear, anxiety, and doubt float by. Feel the deep, quiet strength that pervades your entire being.

When you are ready, take a few deep breaths. As you breathe, consciously infuse your body with a heightened sense of vitality…infuse your mind with clarity and calm…fill your heart with warmth, tenderness, and appreciation for yourself and the world you live in. Carry this feeling with you and allow it to pervade and energize your next activity.

2 FLOW SEQUENCE ▼ ▼ ▼

ACCESS

Pause,
Become aware of your surroundings.
Feel where your body touches the world.
Bring your awareness to the weight and warmth
where your body touches your own body.

As you breathe,
exhale long and slow,
softly sigh as though releasing a heavy load.
Let go into gravity.
Allow the inhalation to come naturally,
effortlessly receive the breath.

Scan your body for signs of tensions.
Breathe your awareness into those regions.
As you exhale, soften and open around the tension. Smile to yourself.
Gently remind yourself.
"I don't need to hold this in my body."

After scanning and releasing throughout your whole body,
allow all sensations to flow within the space of your
awareness; experience the symphony of life resonating within your body.
Remember—there is space for all sensations within your experience.

If tension or pain still remains, soften around it.
Allow the sensations to float freely and to change *without resistance.*
Gently bring your awareness to the flow of thoughts, feelings,
and images in your mind.
Simply notice (without commentary) how they change from
moment to moment.
Attend to the *process* of change without concern for the particular
content of the thoughts and images.

If you notice your attention tightening
around any thought, feeling, image, or sensation,
simply notice the gripping,
smile to yourself,
breathe into it,
and let it flow.

APPRECIATION

Now, simply rest in the flow.
Remember—there is space for *everything* within your experience.
Resistance is pain.
Trust gravity.
Relax into the flow…
Allow your awareness to become subtler with each breath.
Appreciate the resonant quality of the flow state.
Practice fine-tuning and returning to this resonant flow state.

REENTRY AND EXPRESSION

Once again,
become aware of your contact with the world around you.
With eyes closed, sense the space around you.
Sense how the surrounding space connects you to everything.
Experience the sounds, smells, and feelings filling this space.

As your eyes gently open,
allow them to be soft and receptive.
See without *looking*.
Aware of breath…
Aware of gravity…
Aware of the resonance…
of free flowing life within you.
Carry the calm vitality of this experience into action.

CULTIVATION OF FLOW

Human circuitry is remarkably sensitive to change. It requires frequent fine-tuning to maintain peak performance.

Life will inevitably challenge you.

Monitor your stress levels throughout each day. By consciously recognizing and reducing the "noise" in your life, an underlying harmony naturally begins to emerge.

Patient, persistent practice pays off. If you have thirty seconds at a stoplight or thirty minutes at lunch or after exercise, use it to fine-tune your system. Even if some tension still remains afterward, give yourself credit for what you let flow. We each come fully equipped with everything we need to learn about how to relax. Perhaps no one has ever showed you how to access these potentials.

With practice, you will notice some wonderful changes in your body, mind, and performance.

FREE FLOW: TEN SIMPLE STEPS
FOR MASTERING STRESS

The following ten steps will guide you through the basic stages of the previous technique. Once you understand this basic outline you will have a simple, quick, and effective stress method for recognizing and reducing symptoms of stress before they can accumulate.

1. Pause, and relax into a comfortable position with spine straight.
2. Become aware of your surroundings.
3. Breathe awareness into your body. Exhale long and slow, sighing, *ahh*...trust gravity.
   Allow inhalations to fill you effortlessly.
4. Scan your body for signs of tensions.
5. Smile tenderly to yourself, remembering, "I don't need to squeeze so tightly."
6. Open and gently soften around any tension or pain.
7. Eyes soft, jaw relaxed, arms heavy and warm, mind at ease, rest and be energized by the release of free-flowing life around you.
8. Picture in your mind your next activity and imagine carrying this feeling of ease and energy into action.
9. Gently open your focus to be aware of the space around you.
10. Carry this calm vitality into action.

Experience this free flow at work. Share it with others.

3 RELAXING THE BODY ▼ ▼ ▼

1. Select a comfortable place to sit or lie down. Remove your shoes, loosen your belt or tight clothing. Stretch out on your back, arms resting by your sides, feet slightly apart, eyes gently closed.
2. Think, "Now I am going to relax completely. When I finish I will feel fully refreshed and energized."
3. Bring your attention to your feet, wiggle your toes, flex your ankles.
   Then *let go*, release all the tension, and let your feet rest limp and heavy.
4. Bring your attention to your legs, your knees and thighs, up to your hips.
   Imagine them just sinking into the floor or chair, heavy and relaxed.
5. Bring your attention to your arms, elbows, and upper arms, all the way up to your shoulders.
   Imagine all the tension just melting away.
6. Bring your attention to your abdomen.
   Let the tension go, and allow your breathing to flow more smoothly and deeply.
7. Bring your attention to your stomach and chest, up to your throat and neck. As you continue breathing more deeply, just imagine all the tension flowing out as you are relaxing more and more deeply.
8. Now, bring awareness to your throat, neck, and head, feeling loose and relaxed.
   Relax your facial muscles.
   Let the jaw drop, parting the lips and teeth.
   Picture yourself completely relaxed.
9. If you are aware of any remaining tension anywhere in the body, mentally go to that area and allow tension to release and dissolve away.

10. Continue to remain in this completely relaxed state for five to ten minutes. You may picture pleasant thoughts, or simply blank your mind and enter a state of light sleep.

11. When you are ready to get up, say to yourself, "I have been deeply relaxed. I am now ready to awaken, feeling completely refreshed, energized and relaxed."

12. Begin to move by flexing the ankles, wiggling the toes.
    Then wiggle the fingers, and gently shake your wrists.

13. Bend the right knee, and then the left knee.
    Bend the right arm and then the left arm.

14. Open your eyes. Stretch each arm over your head.
    Then slowly sit or stand up, and stretch again.

You are now ready to continue with your activities.

4 BODY SCAN ▼ ▼ ▼

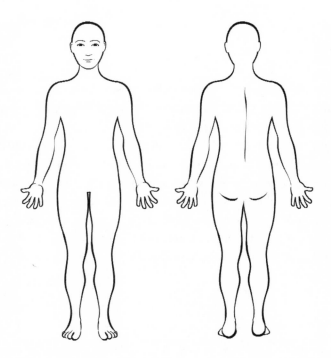

This body-scan technique will help you reclaim the all too often "lost world" of your body. With continued use of this charting technique and frequent mental scans throughout the day, the richness of physical sensual aliveness will continue to reveal itself to you, and the warning signs of stress will be quickly recognized.

Indicate intensity of sensations in any region in the illustrations above on a scale of -5 to +5, 0 being neutral, -5 extreme discomfort, and +5 extreme pleasure. Doodle in the feelings of tingling, vibration, density, numbness, and so forth. Do not draw conceptualized anatomical structures (bones, organs, etc.). Graphically represent feelings in any region you have awareness of.

You may wish to make a photocopy of this page.

5 AUTOGENIC IMAGERY ▼ ▼ ▼

This practice is particularly effective for bringing harmony to your mind-body. It uses a special sequence of phrases or formulas that directly affect the control systems of your body.

Begin by assuming a comfortable position. Keep your body still and comfortable. Take five slow, full breaths inhaling and exhaling through both nostrils. Then begin to breathe slowly and smoothly with no pause between exhalations and inhalations. Gently concentrate your attention on the sensations of breath flowing past the tip of your nostrils. If your mind wanders, gently bring it back to the space between the nostrils. Continue now to breathe slowly and easily without having to strain to get more air.

IMAGES FOR QUIETING THE BODY

Now, as you silently repeat or listen to the following phrases, effortlessly allow yourself to visualize, imagine, and feel the flow of relaxation pervading your entire body. Simply allow the body to respond to these world-images:

I feel quiet...
I am beginning to feel quite relaxed...
my feet, my ankles, my knees, and my hips feel heavy, relaxed, and comfortable...
the whole central region of my body feels relaxed, and quiet...
my hands feel heavy, warm, and relaxed...
my arms and my shoulders feel heavy, relaxed, and comfortable...

my neck, my jaw, and my forehead feel deeply relaxed.
They feel comfortable and smooth...
my whole body feels quiet, comfortable, and deeply relaxed...

IMAGES FOR QUIETING THE EMOTIONS

Continue now to remain comfortable and relaxed as you visualize, imagine, and feel the following phrases for calming your emotions and infusing your body with warmth:

My arms and hands are heavy and warm...
I feel quiet, very quiet...
my arms and hands are relaxed, relaxed and warm...
my hands are warm...
warmth is flowing into my hands, they are warm...very warm...
my hands are warm...relaxed and warm...
as I breathe I am filled with warmth and well-being...
exhaling I am able to let my heart and mind open to allow
my feelings to come and flow...

IMAGES FOR QUIETING THE MIND

With each phrase, imagine and *feel* a growing internal quietness and heightening of internal attention:

I feel quiet now...
my mind is very quiet, calm and clear...
as I withdraw my thoughts from the surroundings and I feel serene,
still, and at ease...
deep within myself
I can visualize and experience myself as relaxed, comfortable,
open, flowing, and still...
I am alert in an easy, effortless, quiet, inward-turned way...
my mind is calm, clear, and quiet...

I feel an inward quality of stillness and quiet.
Energizing the mind and body

When you are ready to move into action, imagine and affirm the following phrases as you stretch your body:

I feel rested and reenergized now...
I can feel life energy flowing through my arms and hands...
I feel life energy moving and flowing
through my face, and pervading my arms, chest, and abdomen,
   my legs and lower body...
my whole body feels energized, enlivened, unified, and wholly alive...
my mind is calm, clear, and alert...
I feel alert, enlivened, and ready for action.

When you're ready, stretch, breathe, and allow your eyes to gently open.

6 CREATING AN INNER OASIS ▼ ▼ ▼

Sit or position yourself comfortably and draw your attention inward. Allow outer sounds and movements to come and go without distraction. Now, allow your inner vision to draw you to a special place of beauty, peace, or power that represents an idealized environment or atmosphere for your deep relaxation and reenergizing. This may be a scene from your memory or imagination, or a composite image of both fantasy and reality. It should be a quiet environment, perhaps by the seashore, in the mountains, or even in your own backyard.

Allow this image to come alive for you now. Vividly imagine with all your senses that you are actually here alive in this experience. As you breathe, energize all of your senses. Vividly see the shapes and colors around you. Hear the sounds in the environment around you. Smell the fragrances in the air, and taste any wonderful flavors that are a part of this vision. With your body, feel the temperature of the air or breeze, and sense the shapes and textures of the world around you here. And spatially sense yourself amid your surroundings, being aware of what is above you, behind you, in front of you, and to either side.

Rest here now. Heal, harmonize, and come to rest.

Allow each breath to infuse you with calm, power, clarity, and peacefulness—whatever feelings you most need. Allow your mind to absorb the peacefulness and natural vitality of this wonderful place. Experience or imagine your body and mind as whole and complete. Imagine and sense your body-mind coming into a perfect harmony and resonance with the healing and energizing qualities of this special place of beauty, peace, and strength.

Rest here now. Absorb whatever qualities or energies you most need. Allow yourself to be attuned to a state of perfect harmony and resonance.

When you are ready, gently allow this image to melt into openness within you. Carrying with you all of the energy, vitality, beauty, power, peace, serenity, and strength of this mental oasis, become aware of your surroundings. As you breathe, imagine that you are receiving inspiration from this place within you. As you move into action, feel as though these positive feelings are welling up within your mind and body, and flowing into your outer life and actions. Let your outer world reflect some of the special qualities of your inner oasis.

7 RAINBOW LIGHT RELAXATION ▼ ▼ ▼

Begin by sitting comfortably, with your spine straight, your eyes soft, jaw loose, and body relaxed. Now vividly imagine that you are surrounded by a luminous mist of relaxation and well-being. Mentally give this mist a red color* and a warm comforting emotional feeling. Next, begin a cycle of five deep and slow breaths. As you inhale this relaxing mist and hold the breath for a slow count of five, imagine it filling your head, neck, and shoulders and soaking deeply into every pore and fiber of your head, neck, and shoulders. As you breathe out, imagine exhaling all of your physical tensions, thoughts, cares, or mental dullness that may be stored in this region of your body. Imagine exhaling any physical, emotional, or mental disease as smoke or fog being flushed completely out of your body by this luminous relaxing mist. Imagine this fog or smoke dissolving completely into the space around you.

With a second cycle of five breaths, focus upon your torso, including your hands and arms. Vividly imagine and feel this relaxing mist flowing in through your nostrils, filling the center of your chest, and then spreading throughout your hands, arms, and torso, filling this region completely with a luminous, warm, relaxing feeling of red mist and light. As before, hold the first breath for a slow count of five, allowing the oxygen to saturate and nourish your tissues and wash away the waste products from your muscles

* Different colors may subtly influence different effects for different people at different times. Once you have mastered the basic visualization, experiment with imagining different colors to determine what frequency of the mental spectrum works best for you. If you find it difficult to visualize colors, begin by looking at an appropriately colored piece of paper, foil, or film, or at a spectrum of sunlight cast on a wall by a crystal. With practice this technique will become both simple and powerfully effective.

and brain. Vividly imagine that this entire region is now alive with a vital-
izing red glow of deep relaxation.

With a third cycle of five breaths, direct your attention to your lower
body, including your hips, buttocks, genitals, legs, and feet. As you inhale,
vividly imagine this luminous relaxing mist flowing down to your navel, and
as you exhale, imagine it diffusing to completely fill the whole lower portion of your body. Allow the muscles and tissues to be oxygenated and
cleansed. Allow the following breaths to find their own natural rhythms
and depth. Vividly sense and imagine this entire region of your body aglow
with a deep, soothing sense of relaxation, warmth, and vitality.

With a last cycle of five breaths, vividly imagine that you are breathing
in a pure crystalline mist and rainbow-like light. Allow the waves of the
breath to come and flow effortlessly at their own natural rhythm. Imagine
that this luminous substance flows first to the center of your chest and then
pours forth throughout your whole body. Direct this powerful purifying
and harmonizing light to any region of your body that is out of balance and
calls for healing. Sense and deeply feel that your whole being is now pure
and clear like a crystal body that is flooded by rainbow light. Like brilliant
light pouring through a crystal, imagine this luminous energy pouring
through you and out into the world. Imagine that as you mentally direct it
to others this light helps to dissolve their tensions, calm their minds, and
open their hearts to a greater sense of relaxation, warmth, and well-being.
Vividly sense and affirm that this energy and light that pours through you
brings greater harmony to the world in which you live. This becomes a very
simple, very quiet yet powerful gift or blessing that you offer to the world.

You will find that the more vivid your multisensory imagery, the more
powerful and effective will be your use of visualization techniques on your
own mindbody, on the minds and bodies of others, and on the world in
which you live. If it is difficult for you to imagine seeing and feeling the colors and mist, energize your practice with a strong sense of confidence and
conviction that it is happening all the same. As you become familiar with
this basic technique, energize and enhance your practice by giving the luminous mist a soothing fragrance, a pleasing sound, and even a soothing or
pleasing taste.

Once you are familiar with this basic technique, you will be able to access
the same results with only four breaths: With the image of red light, draw

in one breath to fill and cleanse your head and neck, one breath to the torso, one to the lower body, and a fourth breath to flood your whole crystal-clear body with rainbow light. With further practice, you will be able to master this method with a single breath by simply supercharging your whole mind-body with a rainbow-like relaxation at any time or place that you wish.

Many of us are more familiar with the symptoms of tension than those of relaxation. Listed below are some frequent indicators of relaxation. Which ones are familiar to you? What others might you add to your list?

I know that I'm relaxed when I experience:

heaviness

lightness

warmth

tingling

yawning

sighing

breathing slower

breathing easier

belly-breathing

openness

connectedness

calm

quiet

peacefulness

flow of feelings

emotional release

quivers

eyes softening

muscles softening

PART TWO

▼ ▼ ▼ **CONCENTRATION**

With an eye made quiet by the power
of harmony and the deep power of joy
we see into the heart of things.
William Wordsworth

FOCUSING THE MIND ▼ ▼ ▼

The moment one gives close attention to anything,
even a blade of grass, it becomes a mysterious, awesome,
indescribably magnificent world in itself.

Henry Miller

L ife is learning. The amount of real learning that takes place is directly
proportional to our ability to concentrate or focus our attention on any
one thing for a period of time. But real learning is not just the acquisition
of knowledge, but the ability to penetrate deeply into the meaning behind
superficial knowledge.

By developing our ability to concentrate, we develop our capacity to
integrate related thoughts, facts, and information into a structural frame-
work that reveals a deeper, more synthesized meaning than that which is
immediately apparent to the superficial or unconcentrated observer. The
concentrated mind enables us to accelerate our growth and learning because
it provides us with direct access to knowing and to understanding the mean-
ings and causes underlying ordinary appearances.

For most people, the distracted and uncontrolled circulation of thoughts
and mental impressions, or the narrow-minded preoccupation with certain
aspects of these impressions, is the norm. These distracted and confused
states of mind do not lead to peak performance or creative insight. From its
usual vantage point of discursive thought or casual observation, our unfo-
cused mind does not have the stability or power to pierce the veil of superficial appearance and to directly perceive the deeper levels of meaning and

the underlying interrelationships to which all great scientists and philosophers refer.

The father of the modern psychology of consciousness, Dr. William James, was once asked how long it was possible to sustain a focus of concentration upon a single object. After some reflection, he replied that to the best of his knowledge or ability, four seconds was the maximum. For most of us, even that would be a feat! Yet, as we explore the literature on peak performance from the world's great contemplative traditions, we find descriptions of and directions for systematically developing states of concentration and stabilized attention for periods of minutes, hours, even days without distraction.

We have all had a taste of concentration. At different times in our lives, each of us has fully given our attention to a loved one, a beautiful sunset, a resounding symphony, or a project that completely absorbed us. And it is possible to train our minds to increase and develop such concentration.

Often cited as the initial indicator that one's practice of concentration is becoming stable is that one's attention can stay unbroken on the count of 7, then 21, then 108 breaths. As this concentration grows, even when our attention does wander, the distraction is immediately recognized and we can return our mind to the object of concentration.

In the next phase, concentration matures to become contemplation. Here, we begin to experience a sense of connectedness, a flow, between ourself the observer and the object of our attention. Finally, at the third stage of unification, we have wholeheartedly and uninterruptedly given our attention to our object. Here, we enter into an intimate relationship with it, knowing it intuitively as though it were one with us. You may have spontaneously experienced this quality of complete concentration sometime when you were in love or when your attention was completely captured by something of inspiring beauty.

With practice, our minds will grow more stable, and our perception of ourselves and our world will gradually change. New domains of intuitive understanding will be revealed and incorporated into our lives. Our sense of isolation will diminish and we will feel an interrelatedness, an empathy, compassion, and respect—for ourselves, each other, and the world.

Developing strong concentration is similar to developing physical strength. The patient, persistent practice that the following techniques bring will certainly build your ability to concentrate. Once this skill is developed, a concentrated beam of awareness can be focused upon any activity, leading to a deeper understanding and appreciation of ways to enhance your perception and performance.

As you proceed, remember the following advice:

▼▼ Be patient with everyone, but above all with yourself. I mean do not be disheartened by your imperfections, but always rise up with fresh courage. How are we to be patient in dealing with our neighbor's faults if we are impatient in dealing with our own? He who is fretted by his own failings will not correct them. All profitable correction comes from a calm and peaceful mind.

Saint Francis de Sales

GUIDELINES FOR DEVELOPING
CONCENTRATION SKILLS ▼ ▼ ▼

Before an instrument can be used it must be created. It is true that most of us learn to concentrate on worldly affairs, but all such effort is directed towards the analysis, synthesis and comparison of facts and ideas, while the Concentration which is a necessary prelude to Meditation aims at unwavering focus on the chosen thing or idea to the exclusion of any other subject...complete one-pointedness of thought upon the subject in hand, be it a pencil, a virtue, or a diagram imagined in the mind.

Christmas Humphreys

1. SELECTING AN OBJECT/FOCUS OF CONCENTRATION

There are literally thousands of objects of attention that have been prescribed for developing concentration. Some ancient traditions would emphasize concentration upon divine attributes such as strength, power, compassion, beauty, or mercy. Others recommend contemplation on the gross and subtle elements of earth, water, fire, air, and space. Some systems emphasize focusing upon various centers within the body, or upon sacred objects, symbols, or prayers.

The simplest and most direct method for developing mental stability and concentration is to focus upon one's own breath. It is easily found, always present, and self-renewing—approximately at a rate of 21,000 times every day! It is certainly the most effective method for people with busy minds and excessive internal dialogue.

Our state of mind and flow of breath are very closely connected. You can observe for yourself the changes in your own rate and flow of breath when you are feeling anxious, angry, joyful, loving, stressed, or at peace. Simply by bringing our attention to the respiratory process, the mind moves toward greater calm, clarity, and equilibrium.

If you are physically oriented, you might find that some simple movement will help you develop a continuity of concentration. Some martial art form, a gesture or mudra repeated over and over, a yoga posture, or even jogging and cycling can help you begin to develop the initial stages of concentration, if you engage in it wholeheartedly.

If you have a devotional orientation, an object of special meaning can serve well in the development of single-pointed concentration. Choose a picture of a source of inspiration or a sacred symbol or object. The repetition of a short mantra, or the contemplation of some divine prayer or aspect may also be a powerful means to wholeheartedly focus your attention.

The breath, however, can be used at the beginning of these sessions to settle you easily into a quiet state of mind. And it would be ideal to end periods of movement with a few moments of watching the breath.

The breath can become a good friend, a reminder to awaken to the nature of our experiences. With the awareness of a single breath we can focus our attention in the moment, release the tensions of our mindbody and move toward greater harmony.

2. THE KEY TO DEVELOPING CONCENTRATION

Once you start to learn to concentrate, you will find that your mind will sway between holding too tightly and too loosely to its object. It is important to find the balance between these two.

So, once you have settled your mind on your object, and you are focusing your attention, relax your mind a little. If you grasp too tightly at your object, your mind will become agitated and your body tense. If you relax too much, however, your attention will wander or fade.

With practice and patience, you will learn to distinguish between these two states of attention and to deepen your concentration.

3. HOW LONG SHOULD I PRACTICE?

In the beginning it is recommended to keep your sessions short. Frequent short sessions will in the long run be more beneficial and effective than fewer long ones. If your sessions are too long and you push too hard, you will become tired and frustrated.

Let your practice sessions be like the visit of a dear friend—if they leave before you are tired of them, you look forward to their return. If you approach each session with joy, you will have the enthusiasm to practice focusing your attention, and inevitably it will become stable.

The greater your strength of concentration in your practice sessions, the greater will be your power to focus on what you are doing throughout the day.

▼▼ Wisdom is the harmony between our mind and the laws of reality. Morality is the harmony between our convictions and our actions. Concentration is the harmony between our feelings, our knowledge, and our will, the unity of all our creative forces in the experience of a higher reality.

Lama Govinda

See *Guidelines for developing relaxation skills* on pp. 16–26 for further advice.

1 SELF-REMEMBERING ▼ ▼ ▼

If the heart wanders or is distracted, bring it back to the point quite gently...and even if you did nothing during the whole of your hour [of contemplation] but bring your heart back, though it went away every time you brought it back, your hour would be very well employed.

Saint Francis de Sales

As you read these words, know that you are reading. Developing our ability to be aware of what we are doing is called self-remembering. This practice enables us to fine-tune our perceptions and actions. It brings calm, clarity, and freedom to the mind, qualities that are necessary for recognizing the limiting patterns of habitual thought and actions, and for choosing more creative and effective options. With this awareness we can guide our lives toward attaining the goals we wish to reach. For example,

▼▼ Beginning, I am aware of beginning.
Reading, I am aware of reading.
Breathing in, I know I am breathing in.
Breathing out, I know I am breathing out.
Listening, I know I am listening.
Touching, I know I am touching.
Lifting, I am aware of lifting.
Sitting down, I am aware of sitting down.
Thinking, I am aware of thinking.
Experiencing fear, I am aware of feeling fear.

Experiencing joy, I am aware of feeling joy.
Intending, I am aware of intending.
Finishing, I am aware of finishing.

Practice this when you:
Simply go for a walk.
Simply listen to music.
Simply eat a meal.
Simply read.

Above all, *keep your mind wholeheartedly on what you are doing*. And when it wanders—as it surely will—simply bring it back to what you are doing, and without self criticism or lecturing yourself, return to your practice of self-remembering.

2 AN ANTIDOTE TO DISCOURAGEMENT ▼ ▼ ▼

I t is easy to feel that a practice session has been a waste of time when much of it is taken up with distraction or agitation. A simple remedy to this, and a way to help develop your concentration, is to break up your hour or half-hour or less into many smaller sessions with very short breaks in between. (Also, you could apply this method anytime you have a few moments to spare.)

1. Sit comfortably with the spine straight.
2. Gently and completely exhale.
3. As you exhale, softly vocalize the sound *Ahhh*. Allow the sound to open and flow outward. Allow your mind to open and flow with the sound as one continuous wave of awareness, until it reaches the moment when distraction or agitation arises.
4. At the first sign of distraction or agitation, immediately stop the session.
5. Relax, take a break for 15–20 seconds. Look around, stretch your legs if you like, then repeat steps 2–5.

Repeat these steps as many times as you like within the time you have allowed for your session. Gradually you will become accustomed to these short spans of continuous attention and applied concentration. Initially your concentration will last for only a few seconds, but with practice you will develop stability, and the depth and duration of your concentration will grow.

As your concentration develops, consciously feel that your mind and the sound of *Ahhh* are continuously opening outward, even when you stop the *Ahhh* to take another breath.

▼▼ The temple bell stops
But I still hear the sound
coming out of the flowers.

Basho

3 ZEN BREATHING EXERCISE ▼ ▼ ▼

As concentration and attention increase, the mind becomes clear and balanced. More and more sharply we see how things are changing in each instant, how these are ultimately not a source of lasting happiness, and how the whole mindbody process flows according to certain laws (karma) empty of any permanent self.... These profound insights become clear simply from increasing mindfulness, penetrating awareness of our own process. With these insights wisdom arises, bringing equanimity, loving-kindness and compassion, for in experiencing the emptiness of self we see the unity of all beings.

Jack Kornfield

1. Sit comfortably with your spine straight. Establish a proper motivation for beginning the session.
2. Bring your attention to either the sensation of breath flow at the tip of your nostrils or your abdomen, as you inhale and exhale naturally.
3. Consciously take a few deep breaths, but do not strain. Simply emphasize the movement in order to clarify the sensations that you are attending to.
4. Now, allow the breath flow to find its own natural rhythm. Allow the body to breathe without interference. Allow the inhalations and exhalations to come and go, effortlessly keeping a keen awareness of the process.
5. Gently and unwaveringly allow your attention to float on the changing rhythms of your in-breath and out-breath. Whenever your attention wanders or becomes diffused—and it quite often will—gently but firmly bring your awareness back to the breath.

Initially, it may be helpful to count your breaths with each exhalation up to ten. When you reach ten, start your count again. If your attention is distracted, or fades out, begin at one again. The aim is not to arrive anywhere but to develop the capacity to be fully present in each moment, one after another.

Don't be discouraged or disheartened by distractions or mental dullness. This is to be expected. With practice, you will be able to catch the distractions and bring your attention back to the breath. Eventually your concentration will stabilize, and even though distraction will still arise, you will be able to stay unwaveringly upon your object of concentration. You will have developed the capacity to bring a continuum of undistracted, deeply penetrating attention to whatever field of perception or contemplation you choose.

The force of the mind, and its illuminating, penetrating capacity, once it is developed, is similar to the power and coherence of a laser beam compared to the flickering candle of our ordinary distracted states of consciousness. This power and clarity of the finely tuned mind is one of the most useful tools that a human being can develop.

▼▼ When meditation is changed from the breath to awareness of change, the teacher instructs the meditator with a specific formula for beginning the practice of sweeping the attention through the body, part by part, feeling the impermanence of all touch and sensation. As the awareness of impermanence continues, the meditator will see how the power of his concentration and mindfulness can unblock the flow of energy in the body, the sweeping becomes more rapid and more clear. As the body becomes clear for the flow of energy and the impermanence and change of all sensations becomes more apparent, the focus of attention of the meditator moves to the region of the heart. Now mindfulness and concentration on the changing sensations and feelings are so strong that all sensations, even the movement of mind, are experienced as changing, as vibrations. Perception of the whole world, matter and mind, becomes reduced to various levels of vibration in a constant state of change. The meditator continues to apply his understanding and growing skill and applies his penetrating insight to directly experiencing the true nature of existence.

U Ba Khin

4 SUFI BREATHING EXERCISE ▼ ▼ ▼

There is One Holy Book, the sacred manuscript of nature, the only scripture which can enlighten the reader.... It is when the eye of the soul is opened and the sight is keen that the Sufi can read the divine law in the manuscript of nature.

Hazrat Inayat Khan

The following series of Elemental Purification Breaths come to us through one of the lineages of Sufi teachings. This is a perfect focusing and centering practice to begin your day, and takes only the time of twenty-five breaths. It can be used as a short and simple meditation practice in itself, or as a warm-up concentration exercise to focus the mind for another meditation practice you may choose to do.

Begin by breathing naturally in and out through your nostrils for five full breath cycles. This first series of five breaths is focused on purifying yourself with the element of earth. As you inhale, imagine that you draw the energy and magnetism of the earth up into you. It circulates through your subtle energy systems and replenishes and renews the vitality and strength of your body. As you exhale, imagine that the magnetic field of the earth draws all the heavy, gross elements or energies within you down into the ground to be purified and released. With each breath, you feel revitalized, lighter, less dense, and clearer to the free flow of breath, life, energy.

Then with a second series of five breaths, imagine purifying yourself with the energy of water. Inhaling through your nose and exhaling through your mouth, envision a waterfall of pure, clear energy pouring down into you from the heavens above, flowing through you, and dissolving, purifying anything within you that might block the flow of life-energy moving through you. With each breath, you are washed clean and clear, as this stream of energy and light flows through you.

With the next series of five breaths, purify yourself with the element of fire. Inhaling through your mouth and exhaling through your nostrils, let the breath flow focus at your solar plexus as you inhale, and then rise up and radiate as light from your heart-center, shining out between your shoulder blades, and like a fountain of light up through the crown of your head. Inhaling fire, exhaling light, envision and affirm that this circulation of energy is a purifying fire gathering any remaining impurities or congestion and burning them into radiance and light in the fires of your heart.

With the next cycle of breaths, imagine purifying yourself with the air element. Inhaling and exhaling through your mouth, imagine the air element sweeping through you like the wind blowing through the spaces of your whole body, purifying any sense of density or obstruction that may remain.

Finally, breathing very gently through your nostrils, envision yourself being purified by the most subtle element—the "ether" element of the ancients, or the most subtle energies that infuse space, or the quantum field of infinite potentials. Let this most subtle breath dissolve any remaining sense of solidity or density and let your heart and mind open to be clear and vast like the infinite sky.

Energized and purified, sense the subtle, yet profound shift that has taken place in the course of only twenty-five breaths. Carry the sense of focus, calm, and deep connectedness from this practice into your next meditation or into your daily life.

5 BREATHING EASY▼ ▼ ▼

Sit comfortably and relax, and bring your awareness to your breathing. As you breathe out, naturally dissolve and let go of all the negative energy that you wish to be free from. As you breathe in, allow the breath to naturally and effortlessly fill you with the positive qualities you want to be energized by. Allow the breath to fill you as a natural reflex to the deep exhalation.

Think of a word that reflects the quality you wish to be filled with—for example, *relaxing, harmonizing, balancing, energizing, peace, patience*. See that particular quality as luminous energy that, as you inhale, rises within you, fills you and flows through you, completely permeating your body-mind. Allow this light energy to dissolve all your negative states of mind, tension, or pain. Allow the natural vitality of life to awaken within you.

As you exhale, say to yourself *dissolving, melting, releasing*, or *letting go*. Feel the tensions, thoughts, cares, and painful states of body-mind flowing out of you and melting away. Emphasize the long, slow exhalation; then allow the inhalation to come naturally, effortlessly.

Place your hands on your belly and quietly breathe in and out. Allow your belly to gently rise and fall as the breath flows through you.

After a few minutes, allow the breath, after naturally filling your belly, to rise up to the center of your chest and fill you as though a bubble of breath were filling you from within. Exhale through an imaginary hole in the center of your chest, and allow your heart to open...

Breathing into your hands...bringing the air up to fill your heart...opening the heart...exhaling...opening and letting go.

6 ABDOMINAL BREATHING▼ ▼ ▼

When under stress, most of us tend to breathe in short, shallow breaths, primarily by expanding our chests. This thoracic breathing is not the most efficient way to breathe. Not only does it prevent the lungs from filling and emptying completely, it can also contribute to increased muscle tension.

During stressful situations, it is especially important that we breathe from our abdomen, not just our chest. Abdominal breathing relaxes the muscles, massages the internal organs, and allows more oxygen to energize our system.

The ideal times to practice abdominal breathing are when you are feeling tense or anxious or in need of energizing your body or calming your mind. Just a few of these complete breaths are wonderfully calming and won't be noticed during a meeting or a phone call. This simple procedure is *very* effective.

1. Sit comfortably with your spine straight.
2. Exhale completely.
3. Inhale very slowly, allowing the breath to enter effortlessly through your nose. At the same time push out your abdomen as though it were a balloon expanding. Move your chest as little as possible.
4. After your abdomen is stretched, allow your chest to expand with air. This fills the middle part of your lungs.
5. Allow your abdomen to pull in slightly, and your shoulders and collarbones to rise. This fills the upper part of your lungs.
6. Gently hold your breath for a few seconds. At this point, every part of your lungs is filled.

7. Slowly begin to exhale through your nose. Breathe abdominally by lifting your diaphragm and allowing your lungs to empty. Proper exhalation releases used air and opens space for fresh air to enter.

Though at first this way of breathing may feel awkward, once you become familiar with the technique it can be done quite easily and comfortably.

7 CONCENTRATION:
THE SIMPLE NINE-PART BREATH ▼ ▼ ▼

As a preliminary to meditation practice, some version or variation of the following concentration technique is recommended. This involves alternating inhalations and exhalations through the left and right nostrils as indicated below. You can either close the opposite nostril with your thumb and index finger or simply focus on one nostril at a time. Do not force or hold the breath, simply allow it to flow deeply, slowly, and at a natural rhythm.

1. Inhale right, exhale left (three times each).
2. Inhale left, exhale right (three times each).
3. Inhale both, exhale both (three times each).

With each inhalation imagine drawing in pure, clear, vital energy in the form of light. Imagine it flowing through you, washing your gross and subtle bodies clean and clear. If you lose track of where you are in the sequence, return to the beginning and start again. Once you become familiar with this basic sequence, even visualizing this breath-flow pattern will be sufficient to bring about the harmonizing and balancing result.

If you have difficulty breathing through your nose due to allergies or congestion, visualizing and imagining that your breath is moving through the nostrils in this way will often be an effective means of clearing your sinuses.

In addition to the image of inhaling pure white light or vital energy, the following visualization is also recommended as a means of further balancing and harmonizing the mindbody:

1. As you exhale through the left nostril, imagine breathing out all your attachment and desire toward ideas, objects, perceptions, or states of mind. Visualize them as dark red in color.
2. As you exhale through your right nostril, imagine breathing out all your anger, resentment, and frustration. Visualize them as smoke.
3. As you exhale through both nostrils, imagine breathing out all your confusion, ignorance, pride, and any other mental state that obscures your perception and understanding of the true nature of yourself and the world around you. Visualize these as darkness.

Each time you inhale, breathe in light. As you exhale, imagine that all your mental and emotional confusions, your darkness and dullness of mind dissolve completely into space, atomized and utterly gone. This is an excellent technique to apply frequently throughout the day, whenever you need to clear and focus your mind. (See: *Balancing breath, brain and mind*, pp. 220–22).

Our discovery of God is in a way God's discovery of us. We know Him in so far as we are known by Him, and our contemplation of Him is a participation in God's contemplation of Himself. We become contemplatives when God discovers Himself in us. At that moment, the point of our contact with God opens up and we pass through the center of our souls and enter eternity.

Thomas Merton

I f you have a devotional orientation, the most effective object for your development of concentration might be a statue or picture of, say, Jesus, Mother Mary, Buddha, a great saint, or a special teacher. Gazing at or visualizing one of these images or even a sacred symbol, or reciting a prayer or mantra, could well be effective as a means for collecting your mind and bringing it to a calm state of concentration.

1. Select an object with special meaning.
2. Wholeheartedly devote your mind and body to this object for a chosen period of time.
3. Whenever your mind wanders, gently return it.
4. When you finish, relax, rejoice, and give thanks.
5. Carry over this calm and clarity into your next endeavor.

Allow yourself to go deeply into your contemplation. As you observe the object of concentration, let your mind settle upon it, relaxed yet alert. As you breathe in and out, feel a flow of energy and information between you and the essence of your object of contemplation. Let your mind move into it. Let its essential nature permeate you and reveal itself to you. Imagine, sense, or feel the essential truth of this image, mantra, sacred symbol, or prayer, and let it resonate deep within you.

▼▼ The most beautiful and most profound emotion that we can experience is the sensation of the mystical. It is the sower of all true science. He to whom this emotion is a stranger, who can no longer wonder and stand rapt in awe is as good as dead. To know that what is impenetrable to us really exists, manifesting itself as the highest wisdom and the most radiant beauty which our dull faculties can comprehend only in their most primitive forms—this knowledge, this feeling, is at the center of true religiousness. My religion consists of a humble admiration of the illuminable superior who reveals himself in the slightest details we are able to perceive with our frail and feeble minds. That deeply emotional conviction for the presence of a superior reasoning power, which is revealed in the incomprehensible universe, forms my idea of God.

Albert Einstein

9 SPHERES OF MIND ▼ ▼ ▼

Before me peaceful
Behind me peaceful
Under me peaceful
Over me peaceful
Around me peaceful

Traditional Navajo Prayer

S it comfortably with your spine straight and your body relaxed. For a
few minutes allow your attention to follow the breath, or do the nine-
part breathing mentioned earlier.

With your eyes closed or slightly open, reach out into the space in front
of you and imagine that you are catching hold of a ball in the palm of your
hand. Bring this imaginary ball closer to you and add a sense of vividness
to its shape and size. Now imagine that in an instant this transforms into a
ball of brilliant white light, three-dimensional, transparent, luminous, and
lacking solidity. Imagine that this ball of light radiates a sense of quiet calm
and well-being. As you breathe, feel this ball of light come to rest at the center of your chest. Rest your attention here, effortlessly. Whenever it wanders, return to the inner visualization of a radiant sphere at the center of
your chest.

If you feel a tightness in your chest when using the image above, or your
mind is too restless to focus, the following variation can be used instead.

Establish the image of a luminous sphere shining at the center of your
chest. Now, regardless of what direction you are actually facing, mentally
orient yourself as though you were facing east. Imagine that this sphere

shoots straight out in front of you, beyond the eastern horizon to a place hundreds, thousands, or millions of miles away. Rest your mind on this sphere in the distant space. Experience the freedom of mind to reach out and extend itself farther and farther without any limitation.

If the mind begins to lose interest or drift off to thoughts, once again establish the image of the radiant sphere at your chest. This time shift your attention to the western horizon behind you and vividly imagine sending the sphere out infinitely far in that direction. Rest your mind there. Again, when the mind wanders, reestablish the image at your heart.

With the next cycle, send the mind-sphere off to the southern direction to your right. Imagine the sphere hovering and radiating light thousands and millions of miles to your right. Allow the mind to rest there undistracted and at ease. As before, when your attention wanders or fades, shift again, this time to focus on a sphere of light in space over the northern horizon to your left. With each phase of this practice, take as long over the visualization as feels comfortable.

Traditionally, you would now continue with the horizon in front of you to your left and right, and then behind you to your left and right, and even above and far below you. In any case, you should simply let the mind rest on this luminous sphere, this extension of your mind going out into the far distance. Spend as much time as you need to get the feeling of the expansive, limitless nature of your mind.

Finally, expand your mind to encompass all the spheres that you have sent out in all directions along with the original one at your heart. Lucidly and effortlessly rest your mind in this experience of simultaneous expansion to all these directions.

The reason for changing directions in this method is to introduce an element of novelty, freshness, and play. Therefore wait until just before you have lost interest in the direction you are focusing on before changing to another. Remember that the purpose of this method is twofold. First, to stabilize, collect, and focus the mind upon what you are doing. Second, to introduce you to the open, luminous, unimpeded nature of your mind. If your mind were limited in its scope, how could it infinitely expand in any direction you choose

The expansive, luminous, knowing quality of your mind is not limited to the ordinary confines of your body and senses. It is unlimited, omnidirectional, and able to reach out into any number of directions in an instant. This method helps you to begin dispelling the misperception of your ordinary limited sense world. Try and do frequent practice with these extraordinary mental muscles at moments throughout the day.

▼▼ At first the meditator feels like his mind is tumbling
like a river falling through a gorge

in mid-course, it flows slowly like
the gently meandering River Ganges

and finally, the river
becomes one with the great
vast Ocean, where the Lights
of Son (self) and
Mother (ground of being)
merge into one.

Tilopa

10 CONCENTRATION
WITH A NATURAL OBJECT ▼ ▼ ▼

In a flash, the violent mind stood still. Within without
are both transparent and clear. After the great
somersault, the great void is broken through.
Oh, how freely come and go
the myriad forms of things!

Han Shan

Many of us have touched a state of deep concentration during our time with nature. Watching the sun rise, a flowing stream, gazing upon a flower, a cloud, or rain drops on a still pool, our minds have become clear, quiet, and deep. At other times, the chirp of crickets, the sound of breaking waves or a babbling brook have washed away our agitation and left us calm and collected.

1. Select a natural object or process.
2. Attend to it wholeheartedly.
3. Open yourself to let it come in to you, to receive its light, sound, vibration, and life into yourself.
4. Open your heart and mind to embrace and be pervaded by it.
5. As you watch, listen, or feel it, enter into a deep, quiet communion with this natural phenomenon. Allow its essential nature and hidden qualities to reveal themselves intuitively.

▼▼ The sense of wonder is based on the admission that our intellect is a limited and finite instrument of information and expression, reserved for specific practical uses, but not fit to represent the completeness of our being.... It is here that we come in direct touch with a reality which may baffle our intellect, but which fills us with that sense of wonder which opens the way to the inner sanctuary of the mind, to the heart of the great mystery of life and death, and beyond into the plenum void of inner space from which we derive our conception of an outer universe that we mistake for the only genuine reality. In other words, our reality is our own creation, the creation of our senses as well as of our mind, and both depend on the level and the dimensions of our present state of consciousness.

Lama Govinda

11 CONCENTRATION
WHILE WALKING ▼ ▼ ▼

One may start practice with a pure concentration exercise and then change to awareness of process. Initially some teachers prefer using a concentration technique to enable the meditator to still his wandering, undisciplined mind. Later they direct this concentration to the mindbody process to develop wisdom. Other teachers attempt to start directly watching the process, by focusing on changing sensations, feelings or thoughts. This approach must still concern itself with the development of mental qualities of tranquility and concentration before any insight will develop. Buddha taught both approaches at different times according to the needs of his students.

Jack Kornfield

Much of our time in any day can be spent walking. This technique can help us to use walking as a means for developing focus and concentration.

1. Count your first five steps, e.g., right (1), left (2), right (3), left (4), right (5).
2. With the next step, begin at one again and count six steps.
3. With the next step, begin at one again and count seven steps.
4. Continue counting in this way, adding one more step each time until you reach ten.
5. Then, begin again, counting your steps from one to five.
6. Repeat the entire sequence up to ten steps as many times as you like.

If you lose track at any point—and you most likely will—begin again at the cycle of five steps.

Note that if you begin on your right foot, the cycles ending in five, six, seven, nine, and ten steps will end on the right foot. Those ending at six, and eight, will end on the left foot. This pattern will reverse with each full cycle.

▼▼ Remember...
When you walk, walk,
and when you run, run.
By all means, don't wobble!

Zen poem

PART THREE
▼ ▼ ▼ **MEDITATION**

Meditation opens the mind of man to the greatest
mystery that takes place daily and hourly; it widens
the heart so that it may feel the eternity of time and infinity
of space in every throb; it gives us a life within the world
as if we were moving about in paradise; and all these
spiritual deeds take place without any refuge into a
doctrine, but by the simple and direct holding fast
to the truth which dwells in our innermost beings.

Shunryu Suzuki

WHAT IS MEDITATION? ▼ ▼ ▼

At the heart of each of the world's great religions is a profound wisdom tradition with inner transformational teachings. While the exoteric religious traditions offer ethical and moral guidelines necessary for harmonizing and aligning our lives with a universal nature and sacred reality, the inner transformational teachings reveal the spiritual core of these traditions. It is within these esoteric traditions that countless methods of meditation have emerged—like stars coalescing out of a great nebula. These inner traditions present methods of meditation that have been carefully refined over the ages.

Taking these teachings to heart, many students ripened within themselves the same fruit of realization discovered by their teachers. Thus, from generation to generation these liberating and illuminating teachings have been passed from countless teachers to students, giving rise to the myriad lineages of spiritual practice. Each carrying with it both unique and universal aspects. The wisdom of these teachings cascades like countless streams flowing from one source down the many sides of a great mountain.

Through practicing these methods and following these paths of meditation, countless practitioners have realized their own awakenings and have affirmed the realizations for themselves. Through subsequent realizations, these methods and techniques have been progressively tested, refined, and elaborated on to form commentaries to original instructions. As these teachings traveled around the globe over time, these cascades of practices and realizations have given rise to the myriad of the world's diverse wisdom traditions—as well as to the inevitable debate among their adherents regarding what the most true path may be.

In the increasingly common dialogue among modern contemplative inner-scientists from different traditions, attention is inevitably drawn to exploring topics such as, "What is it within and across our various teachings that is truly essential and necessary to preserve and pass on?" and, "What is it that is merely the cultural overlay of tradition that may add little value or even obscure the true message and purpose of these teachings?"

At the turn of the twenty-first century we find ourselves the fortunate recipients of myriad meditative methods and streams of contemplative practice that flow to us across countless generations. These inner teachings offer practical, systematic practices that have been tested and refined over millennia, helping countless practitioners from many traditions discover their true nature and realize their highest potentials.

Though challenged countless times by invaders and dynasties of power in the East, the lineages of wisdom teachings have, until recently, flourished widely in Asian cultures. Throughout the ages these cultures have cherished, nurtured, preserved, and encouraged the investigation and cultivation of the potential for the full development and maturation of the human capacity for power, wisdom, love, and creative compassion. In many ways, the preservation of the Eastern meditative traditions has helped to inspire the rebuilding of Western spiritual and contemplative traditions.

For the first time in history we have access to teachings and teachers from virtually all of the world's great wisdom traditions. While the sheer diversity of traditions can be at times overwhelming, it is also profoundly inspiring, especially when one is able to recognize the common, universal themes that weave across all of the contemplative traditions. By understanding the universal ground of these teachings, their richly diverse methods can be better appreciated and applied to realize the goals of the practices.

▼▼ Mothers of Lineage Masters,
Who have nurtured me with kindness through countless years,
And given fully of your milk of wisdom—
Will the flow of your precious nectar
Now be turned into tears?

Through the power of Interdependent Interrelatedness,
The treasures of Truth you have preserved

And passed on through generations
Survive—
Though you may not.

Through the flower of Interbeing,
And by the Winds of Impermanence,
Your seed is carried across the world
Alive—
And flourishes in fertile, thirsty mindfields
Unknown to you.

Sisters of Niguma, Daughters of Drolma,
My mothers,
Do not despair—
We your foster children,
Whose faces you have never seen,
Will build a living bridge of Dharma,
And dedicate your dream.

                              —*Michelle Levey*
                    From a poem in dedication to the daughters of Tibet

VARIETIES OF MEDITATION ▼ ▼ ▼

Meditation techniques are best understood as methods of mental training, and the goal of meditation is twofold. It involves (1) the conscious cultivation of mental qualities that enhance our understanding, power, and love, and (2) the intentional transformation or lessening of those mind states that block these qualities.

▼▼ Choices in a meditator's life are very simple:
Do those things that contribute to your awareness
and refrain from those things that do not.

Sujata

A person well versed in inner science traditions has access to potent methods for enhancing and developing wholesome and helpful states of mind as well as a veritable apothecary of meditative antidotes to disturbing mental states. Mastering our mind through these methods, we will inevitably develop mastery over our physical and verbal expressions and our relationship with the world.

As we've mentioned, there are thousands of meditation techniques from many different traditions—but all could be classified as belonging to either one or a combination of four categories:

1. concentrative
2. receptive
3. reflective
4. generative

The concentrative approaches to meditation have been described in detail in Part Two of this book. We will now briefly discuss the other three categories.

In contrast to the concentration meditations that narrow and focus the flow of our attention, the methods of receptive meditation teach us to be fully present, mindfully attentive and open to the dynamism, totality, complexity, and subtlety of our experience. Receptive meditations welcome and embrace the flow of all experiences—be they pleasant or unpleasant, inner or outer. In moments when we are enraptured by gazing upon some natural marvel, at times when we give our wholehearted attention to someone, or listen deeply for the answer to our heart's prayer, we catch a glimpse of the mindful presence that is cultivated by the practice of receptive meditation. Traditionally the practices of zazen, mindfulness, dzogchen, mahamudra, self-remembering, and prayer of the heart would be associated with this category. Receptive meditation strengthens our sense of wonder and appreciation, enabling us to effortlessly and precisely attend to the totality of our experience, which is unfolding moment by moment.

The interplay of concentration and receptive meditation allows us to develop the capacity to examine and intuitively understand the deep forces within our ordinary experience. The penetrating insight that develops can then be systematically applied to investigating the very subtle interplay between the phenomena we perceive and the nature of our own mind as the perceiver. As we investigate our participation in the pervasive and dynamic interrelatedness of everything, we will come to sense ourselves as intimately related to and co-creative with the world of our experience.

The practice of reflective or analytical meditation is like disciplined thinking: Choosing a theme, question, or topic of reflection, we focus our reflection, analysis, or contemplation upon it. When our attention wanders to other thoughts, we return to our chosen topic. Traditionally reflective meditation is employed to gain insight into the meaning of life, death, interrelationships, and social conscience, or to come to a conclusive insight regarding some key idea in science, philosophy, or scripture. Following through with our analysis, we arrive at a conclusion giving rise to a strong sense of faith or conviction.

In our day-to-day life, reflective meditation provides us with a powerful and effective tool for focusing our attention upon personal or professional questions in order to discover a creative solution or breakthrough insight. Reflective meditation helps us to understand the issues or inner conflicts that may arise during the practice of other meditations.

Generative meditation practices enable us to consciously cultivate and strengthen specific qualities of mind. Patience, appreciation, sympathetic joy in the well-being of others, gratitude, love, compassion, fearlessness, humility, and tenderness. These qualities, which tend to be associated with aspects of nature, the Divine, or the natural world, are among the attributes that are most commonly cultivated. Generative meditations invite us to actively nurture these strengths of character by thinking, speaking, and acting "as though" these qualities are more fully alive within us.

Properly understood, all of these approaches to meditation are interrelated and mutually enhancing. While the intricacies of these interrelationships are beyond the scope of this book, we simply hope to make clear that the contemplative traditions offer us the inner technology necessary to fulfill virtually any developmental aspiration we may have. Meditation allows us to go beyond words and mental concepts in order to know the true nature and reality of ourselves and our world directly. The pages to come will introduce you to a wide variety of methods to deepen these insights.

MEDITATION TRADITIONS
AS LIBERATIVE ART FORMS ▼ ▼ ▼

As the title of this book suggests, there is a profound aesthetic dimension to the myriad teachings of meditation. The contemplative literature and life stories of many great teachers are replete with examples of their compassionate creativity in transmitting their teachings. Indeed, the teachings of all great teachers may best be regarded as a liberating art form that expresses the realization of the awakened teacher. At the same time, the teachers also skillfully reorganize the attention of their students in a way that transmits to them a glimpse of realization—or at least of its potential.

Robert Thurman, one of our mentors and a professor at Columbia University, expands our understanding of the aesthetic dimension of spiritual teachings: "Upaya, often translated as 'skillful means,' refers to the means by which compassion—the universal compassion of an enlightened being—manifests in actions to enable other beings to find freedom from suffering. That is fundamentally what upaya means…and that word, I think, is best translated as art."

A classic image is that of a finger pointing toward the moon. Here, the moon is what we are being invited to see or discover. It is already there in the sky in all of its beauty and fullness, yet if we just focus on the finger that is pointing we may never see the moon. Similarly, all the teachings on meditation direct our attention toward discovering the deepest, most sublime dimensions of reality that can be realized, or awakened to, in our meditations, yet which defy verbal description.

For example, in one of the Buddha's sermons, though he merely held up a flower and remained silent, he successfully transmitted to his student a profound experience of awakening. At another time, in order to teach his father, the king, he projected from his heart a ray of light that manifested as two buddhas in the sky. Then, from the hearts of each of those buddhas came forth rays of light giving rise to four buddhas, and these then multiplied outward to fill the vastness of the sky with radiant buddha images.

Through parables, teaching stories, inspired poetry and songs, as well as through the simplest of gestures, acts of kindness, or miraculous displays like those of Jesus in the Bible, great teachers have creatively caught and reorganized the attention of their disciples in order to liberate them from their confusions and delusions and to awaken them to a deeper faith and realization of their true nature.

Since each student has a unique constellation of propensities that help or hinder his or her meditation practice, each teacher faces the challenge of intuiting, empathizing, and responding with the most skillful means of instruction to effectively transmit the teachings. In the presence of truly great teachers it is common to hear everyone leaving the meditation hall commenting on how it seemed that the teacher was speaking directly to them and addressing the unique circumstances, struggles, and yearnings at the heart of their own lives.

▼▼ When you search for the guest,
       it is the intensity of the longing
       that does all the work.
       Look at me
       and you will see a slave
       of that intensity!
                      Kabir

MEDITATION:
THE PATH OF AWAKENING ▼ ▼ ▼

One day shortly after his enlightenment, the Buddha was walking
down the road. A man approached reverently and in awe of the
powerful and inspiring presence. Humbly the man inquired, "Are
you a god, come from the heavens to walk among mortal humans
here on earth?" "No," replied the Buddha, "I am not a god."
"Then, are you a magician?" "No," replied the Buddha, "I am not
a magician." "Then who are you?" implored the man. The Buddha
smiled and replied, "I am awake!"

Traditional account of the Buddha

Throughout the ages, countless men and women have awakened to their
true nature. Depending on their culture, language and traditions, they
have been regarded as a buddha, an avatar, the Christ, a saint, a bodhi-
sattva, a wisdom keeper, or a shaman. Each of these individuals had a profound sensitivity to the circumstances and needs of their communities, and
to the skillful means most suited for awakening the individuals to whom
they ministered. The teachings of such people reflect both universal truths
and the societal realities, traditions, worldviews, science, and mythologies
of their times.

The greatest of our teachers have repeatedly reminded us to regard
all the world's great spiritual teachers and teachings as expressions of
a universal compassion that will find its way into the world wherever
the human heart-mind is open. The teachings of all the world's great
religions and great teachers speak universal truths in the particular way

most suited for the people of their place and time.

In the case of Prince Siddhartha, the Buddha—or the "Awakened One"— for forty-five years, he traveled and introduced countless men and women to the inner sciences of awakening. Teaching from a place of profound intuitive wisdom, he, like other great teachers, was able to speak to each person in a way that was intimately attuned to their conditions and help them to awaken more fully. According to some accounts, the Buddha taught 84,000 methods of awakening, while the more mystical traditions say that he taught 84 million methods of awakening. But what is it, you may ask, that the Buddha awakened to? What did he teach others to be awakened to?

First, he taught people to be awake to the far-reaching impacts of their intentions and actions in the world and to bring meditation into action, to be more present and mindful, and to live in a kind and ethical manner.

Second, he taught people how to tame mental and physical energies to develop greater mindfulness and to reduce the mental dullness and agitation that lead to mindless living.

Third, he taught myriad ways to apply mindfulness to the investigation of the nature of reality—through analysis and deep intuition—in order to discover the true nature of all phenomena and the true nature of oneself. There are many levels of awakening to this true nature of reality, and of our selves.

At the first level, we awaken more fully to the frustrations and sufferings of our lives, which have been caused by living in mindless and ignorant ways. This ripens within us a fierce determination to be free of our suffering and evokes a commitment to seeking out methods, teachers, and communities that will support us in our search for true spiritual freedom and happiness.

As our meditations deepen, we awaken to the discovery that everything and everyone is profoundly interrelated, and as our mindfulness of the "interbeing"—to borrow a word from Thich Nhat Hanh—of all beings deepens still more, we awaken to an even greater wisdom and compassion.

As our meditative insights continue to deepen, we awaken to myriad dimensions of our being that are multidimensional and universal. This may happen gradually over time, or suddenly. As we awaken in this way, we come to live in a way that honors the divinity and sacredness that is present as our deepest identity.

▼▼ If you look for the truth outside yourself,
it gets farther and farther away.
Today, walking alone,
I meet him everywhere I step.
He is the same as me, yet I am not him.
Only if you understand it in this way
will you merge with the way things are.

Tung-shan

GUIDELINES FOR
DEVELOPING MEDITATION SKILLS ▼ ▼ ▼

If we—you and I—are to further the evolution of mankind, and not just reap the benefit of past humanity's struggles, if we are to contribute to evolution and not merely siphon it off, if we are to help the overcoming of our self-alienation from Spirit and not merely perpetuate it, then meditation—or a similar and truly contemplative practice—becomes an absolute ethical imperative, a new categorical imperative.... Meditation is simply what an individual at this present stage of average-mode consciousness has to do in order to go beyond that stage in his or her own case.

Ken Wilber

1. CLEAN AND CLEAR SPACE

Create a special space for yourself, either a room or a corner of a room, and use it only for your meditation and heartfelt study or contemplation. Put in this space only those things that help your meditation. Arrange in a pleasing way the pictures and objects that energize the qualities of heart and mind that you are trying to nurture. Arrange a comfortable seat for yourself.

Keep the space clean and clear, as though you were always expecting a special guest. Enter it with respect, and nurture and be energized by the peace, beauty, and healing qualities of it.

2. MINDING THE BODY

In general you will find that it is helpful to precede your quiet sitting meditation with at least a brief period of mindful stretching, tai chi, yoga, or exercise. This will help you to build energy and focus your attention. At times you may find that your mind is simply too agitated to begin with a quiet sitting meditation and that you will gain much greater benefit from a session of walking or moving meditation such as the *Concentration while walking* (pp. 73–74), *Doing what we love to do* (pp. 96–97), or the *Walking meditation* (p. 119).

For sitting meditation, whether you sit cross-legged, in a chair, or kneeling with a meditation bench is largely a matter of style and preference. Experiment and see what works best for you. It is especially important to sit comfortably, with your spine straight and your body upright and relaxed. Sitting in this way it will be much easier to remain alert. Sit naturally and at ease and avoid forcing your body into uncomfortable postures. Your eyes can either be gently closed or softly open—though practicing with them softly open will reduce the tendency to doze off and will help you to carry over the benefits of your meditation into other activities.

With practice you will learn to bring a meditative mind to every activity, whether sitting, standing, walking, or lying down.

3. RELAXATION AND ALERTNESS

We are all familiar with the continuum of arousal—from the deep relaxation of sleep to hyperactivity and alertness. Generally, for most of us, our experience of deep relaxation completely lacks alertness and is at best dull and dreamlike. And at the very height of alertness we are the very opposite of relaxed, experiencing physical tension and mental agitation. Both of these extremes are far from the relaxed yet alert, calm delight of meditative equipoise.

During meditation it is necessary to find the dynamic balance between being too alert—that is, distracted—and too relaxed—that is, dull. Especially in the beginning, much of your session might be spent finding this balance, bringing the mind back from distraction or dullness to a state of relaxed alertness. Eventually, you will become familiar with this state of being. During your meditation sessions you will be able to be deeply relaxed as well as extremely lucid, and during your day-to-day life you will find that your view of the way things are will be less conditioned and obstructed. With this deepening understanding, you will be better able to optimize your response to the challenges and opportunities of each moment with more creative and compassionate attitudes, words, and actions.

4. CONCENTRATION

Concentration is the foundation of meditation. Whatever the technique, it is necessary to have the ability to place your attention on the object of meditation and hold it there without distraction. With patience and practice, your mind will become calmer, more powerful, and able to apply itself to any task with precision and understanding.

As discussed in Part Two, any object or activity can be used for the specific development of concentration. In the following meditations, the same principle applies: Whenever your mind wanders, simply return it to the object of your meditation.

You might find it useful to start your meditation session with a few minutes of one of the concentration techniques, particularly a breathing technique.

5. REFLECTIONS TO ENERGIZE YOUR MEDITATION

Classic texts on meditation offer various reflections to energize and focus the practice of meditation. Here's one series of reflections from the Mahayana tradition.

First, consider the preciousness of your life as a human being, especially as a person who has the freedom and inclination to read a book like this, and the leisure, comfort, and safety to apply yourself to a practice of meditation. Reflect on your extraordinary potential, your capacity to learn and to realize yourself. Reflect also on your access to resources and to the countless helpful conditions that might inspire you on your journey of awakening.

Next, reflect on the reality of change and impermanence. Moment to moment everything in the world around you and the world within you is changing. Sounds, thoughts, pleasures, and pains, the moments and days of your life, the people you love, all come and go. Whatever is born will die, and whatever is created will at some time disintegrate. Taking this to heart, realize that this precious life you live is relatively brief and that it could end at any time. With this in mind, engage in your practice of meditation as a way to accelerate your awakening in order to make the most of the precious moments and days of your life, to realize your highest potentials and help others to do the same.

Next, pause to reflect on the reality of cause and effect, the power of choice and intention in your life. What you experience today is shaped so powerfully by the momentum of your habits and the choices you have made in the past. Be mindful that whatever you choose to pay attention to, and whatever you think, say, or do now will shape your future. Let this awareness inspire you to be mindful of the power behind the choices you make and of the quality of attention you bring to each moment of your life and to your practice of meditation.

Finally, reflect on the potentials you can actualize by freeing your mind from its habits and limitations through the practice of meditation. Not only is it possible to go beyond your stress and confusions, but it is possible to awaken to qualities of being that are profoundly more wise, loving, joyful, peaceful, and powerful than anything you have experienced in the past. Understanding how so much of the suffering in your life and in your world is truly avoidable if you awaken to a deeper wisdom, compassion, peacefulness, and creative compassion, embrace your meditation practice with the discipline and confidence necessary to realize its full potential. To accomplish this for yourself, and in order to inspire and guide others, place your trust in those who can support you and show you the way, and in the teachings and methods that help you on this journey of awakening.

6. TRUST AND REFUGE

We seek a refuge from the chaos and confusion within and around us. Like a child taking refuge in its mother, hikers seeking shelter from a storm, or a person seeking an oasis in a vast desert, we seek sanity in a chaotic world.

Outwardly, we place our trust in the teachers who remind us through their example, their kindness, and their teachings that it is possible to become free from our mental and emotional confusions and to become wise and kind as well. We find strength and guidance in the teachings that show us how to master our minds and find freedom and understanding in our lives. Likewise, we find a refuge in the community of friends and companions who share our study, practice, and investigation of how meditation is practically applied to meeting the challenges and opportunities of daily life.

Inwardly, the teacher reflects the seed of our own potential for deep understanding and genuine kindness. Oral and written teachings point our minds toward the ineffable wisdom that shines like the sun and moves within our hearts, the real mystery that precedes life and endures beyond death. Our companions along the way remind us of the community of people who, from the beginning of time, strove to find the same understanding and preserved and passed the teachings on.

Meditation does not happen in a vacuum, devoid of relationship and sharing with others, whether you are sitting alone in a cave or an office, or meditating in a group. Affirming and trusting your relationships with others and your connectedness with the universe will offer you protection and peace of mind and will inspire your meditation practice.

7. PROPER MOTIVATION

As you begin each session, remind yourself of why you are sitting down to meditate. Why are you giving yourself this gift of time for centering, harmonizing, and fine-tuning? To avoid pain? To be happy? To find peace? To rest or become energized? To commune with the sacred mystery? To awaken to your true nature? To generate loving-kindness and compassion for all beings?

Remember, as you grow in clarity and peace of mind you directly contribute to bringing peace and understanding to others. And remember, as you develop patience toward the people and situations that previously triggered frustration, you will be filling the universe with compassion instead of anger, understanding instead of confusion.

Our intentions reflect back to us an echo of the same energy. How often have you seen actions motivated by fear emphasize the paranoia of a situation? And how often has your love and care touched and opened the heart of another?

Remember, it is not what you do but how and why you do it that really matters. You always have a choice, so use it wisely and creatively.

8. MONITOR YOUR MEDITATION

Your meditation session is likely to go through several phases. Once you have settled down you should stabilize your attention by doing a few moments of a concentration technique. Then you can apply your mind to whatever meditation, either reflective or receptive, you have chosen. Throughout the session, you should use your introspective alertness to monitor the quality of the focus of your attention. In this way you can recognize when your attention has wandered off or faded away. If you find it difficult to stay with the meditation because of too much distraction or dullness, you will find it useful to again do a few minutes of a concentration technique, especially watching the breath. Then, once again you can return to your main meditation.

9. DEDICATION AND SHARING

Take a few moments at the end of each session to consciously extend the positive energies that you have accumulated. Radiate that energy outward as light and love, and imagine it touching others as a vibration that calms, energizes, heals, comforts, and nourishes. Be creative! Imagine you are playing a mental video game. Beam all your positive feelings to your friends, family, people you feel neutral toward, even your enemies. Realize that they all, just like you, want to be happy, want to escape suffering and pain and make the most of their lives. Thus, in your own way, you can make the world a more peaceful place to be in.

In this way, you can see that the time you take to master stress is not selfish. In fact, it is an active form of accepting responsibility for and contributing meaningfully to the lives of others. Though at first these mental training techniques may seem imaginary or conceptual, with practice you will find that you *are* helping—yourself and others.

10. CARRY-OVER PRACTICE

Through your practice of meditation, it is possible to develop many of your previously latent positive qualities. Having used the short time of your quiet meditation to touch and develop the peace, clarity, understanding, kindness, and vitality that is a part of you, you now face the challenge of carrying these qualities into dynamic action as you move through the world. Throughout the day, consciously recall and reenergize these feelings. Particularly when you start to rush and tumble, internally pause and move toward the sense of harmony you experienced earlier in your meditation. Periods of quiet, undistracted meditation are precious opportunities to get in touch with qualities that will gradually grow and pervade even your busiest activities.

You will find that any activity can become an opportunity to train your mind, develop concentration, refine your awareness, or practice kindness. Live in a creative and meditative way, as though your life were a dream and you are busy waking up.

11. CHOOSING A PRACTICE

Your practice of the relaxation and concentration techniques in the previous chapters will greatly aid your meditation. Begin each session with a few minutes of a relaxation or breathing exercise to calm your body-mind—an essential ingredient for successful meditation.

As you become more familiar with meditation, choose the techniques that best suit your temperament and natural inclinations. Remember that each technique is an antidote to a particular difficulty and a means of strengthening certain qualities of mind. If, for example, you have difficulty with anger, then you should meditate on forgiveness (p. 151), loving-kindness (p. 157), and compassion (pp. 154). If you are experiencing physical discomfort or disease, the hollow body meditation (p. 148), meditation on transforming energy (p. 171–72), and pain techniques (p. 217) may be useful. If your mind tends to be tight and narrowly focused, the listening meditation (p. 98), continuum (p. 101), thoughts (p. 108), hollow body (p. 138), and matrix of mind (p. 193) will be helpful to open and relax your mind.

If you are particularly interested in understanding your mind, all of the meditations on pp. 104–10 will be helpful. If you are devotionally inclined, then contemplative practice (p. 66), breathing with all beings (p. 168), meditation on the angel of universal compassion (p. 177), and sphere of light (p. 181) will be fruitful.

Trust your heart and your intuitive sense of what you need, but also understand the importance of being guided by an experienced teacher.

12. THE IMPORTANCE OF A TEACHER

The most effective way to learn anything is to study with someone who has already mastered it. Meditation is certainly no exception. Our mind can be compared to a remarkable musical instrument that is capable of generating the sweetest of music, yet is often plagued with chaotic and noisy sounds. If we sincerely wish to learn to play beautiful music, we must study with a master who knows the instrument inside and out. In order to develop a clear, calm, joyful, and loving mind, we need the guidance of someone who thoroughly understands how the mind works and how it can be transformed.

How do you find a qualified teacher? It is not always so easy. The qualities to look for in a teacher include compassion, knowledge, and insight, morality, sincerity, and skill, both in teaching and in the way they live their life. From your own side, you should have confidence in your teacher and be able to communicate well with him or her. However, don't set out on a frantic guru hunt! Be very discerning; observe carefully; proceed slowly. It may be a matter of years before you meet the person who can answer your questions and be this special kind of friend and mentor.

Meanwhile, you can practice meditations such as those described here and seek the advice of any meditators whose qualities you admire. Learn to trust your own intuitive wisdom, your own inner guru, to tell you whether you are heading toward or away from your goal.

▼▼ Sitting quietly, doing nothing
Spring comes and the grass grows by itself.

Zen poem

▼▼ Meditation techniques are discovered naturally by infants and little children: holding their breath, staring unblinking, standing on their heads, imitating animals, turning in circles, sitting unmoving and repeating phrases over and over until all else ceases to exist. Stop thinking that meditation is anything special. Stop thinking altogether! Look at the world around you as if you had just arrived on Planet Earth. Observe the rocks in their natural formations, the trees rooted in the ground, their branches reaching to the sky, the plants, animals and the interrelationships of each to the other. See yourself through the eyes of a dog in a park. See a flower through its essence. See a mountain through its massiveness. When the mind allows its objects to remain unmolested, there may be no mind and no object—just breathless unity.

Surya Singer

1 DOING WHAT WE LOVE TO DO ▼ ▼ ▼

The first step in growth is to do what we love to do
and to become aware of doing it.

Sujata

What do you really enjoy doing? Have you ever considered that that activity could be an excellent meditation for you? Doing anything we love to do with mindful awareness can be an effective meditation. Meditation is not the activity, but the quality of attention that we bring to the activity. Any activity of our daily life can become a meditation when approached with the intention of developing concentration, clarity, compassion, or insight.

1. Choose an activity you enjoy.
2. Determine that you will bring your full attention to it.
3. Slowly, carefully, and mindfully begin. Remain relaxed, giving your wholehearted attention to what you are doing.
4. Whenever your attention wanders or fades, gently return to being fully aware of what you are doing. If tensions arise, relax and smile playfully to yourself.
5. When the activity or time period that you had designated is over, pause for a few moments to reflect upon the new richness you have discovered in this familiar activity.

In fact, everything that we do throughout the day, even the tasks that we do not like, can become a tool for developing our minds and deepening our concentration.

▼▼ It is a commonly held view that meditation is a way to shut off the pressures of the world or of your own mind, but this is not an accurate impression. Meditation is neither shutting things out nor off. It is seeing clearly, and deliberately positioning yourself differently in relationship to them.

Jon Kabat-Zinn

2 LISTENING ▼ ▼ ▼

At the heart of each of us, whatever our imperfections, there exists a silent pulse of perfect rhythm—a complex of wave forms and resonances which is absolutely individual and unique and yet which connects us to everything in the universe.

George Leonard

Listen...
We are continually hearing information from the world
    around and within us.
Minimize distortion by turning down the volume of your
    internal dialogue.
Imagine that the universe is about to whisper the answer
to your deepest questions...
and you don't want to miss it!

Listen...
Simply, and without analysis or commentary
to whatever sounds enter the sphere of your awareness.
Don't label the sounds.
If you start thinking, remind yourself to just...

Listen...
Effortlessly to sounds.
Let them come to you.
No need to tense or strain.

Trust.
Let go of control. Be at ease.
Still...
quiet...
receptive...
alert...

Listen...
Notice how sounds arise...
and fade away...
Melting into silence or into other sounds.
Don't try to hold them,
allow them to flow...

Listen...
Where do the sounds go? *Listen*...
Where do the sounds come from? *Listen*...
Experience how the space of your awareness
effortlessly accommodates an interpenetrating
symphony of sounds, thoughts, sensations, feelings,
    and visions simultaneously.
Allow, your body-mind to relax
into unencumbered clarity...

Listen...
Allow the answers to these questions to
come as understanding, not as thoughts.

Listen...
And reflect...

Who is listening?

▼▼ The more and more you listen,
the more and more you will hear.
The more you hear, the more and more deeply
you will understand.

Khyentse Rinpoche

3 CONTINUUM ▼ ▼ ▼

There are no ends in life, only processes. Change. Spiritual reality is
physical reality, clearly seen.

Bill Voyd

As you breathe, draw your awareness into this moment. Exhaling, allow
your awareness to flow effortlessly into the next moment. Inhaling,
stabilize and focus your awareness into this moment. Exhaling, feel
the flow of your being unfolding, moving, and continuously expressing itself
through the medium of time and space.

Standing in the present, step into the future and leave the past irretriev-
ably behind you. As you move, feel yourself emanating and moving forward through space and time.

Imagine that as you move you trace a pathway of light and energy
through the fabric of space and time. Imagine that if you turned around you
could actually see this luminous path, like a firefly in the night.

Now, imagine the path you have traced through the world today, during
the past week, the last month. Sense the patterns, cycles, and rhythms of
your goings and comings.

Imagine arising and retracing your steps as you moved around the house,
drove to work or school, dropped into your favorite stores, visited friends,
went for walks or bike rides. See your life as a continuum of light energy patterns unfolding through space and time.

Imagine the pattern of your continuum unfolding since you were born.
Even try to imagine the energy patterns of the body you were in before this
one, and the one before that, and so on, back and back. Really experience

yourself as a dynamic process expressing and unfolding itself through space and time.

Imagine the tons of universal matter that have sustained you and that you have burned as air and water and food during your life's—your lives'—journey.

Imagine your moments of being in love, your experiences of joy, of anger. Feel how your energy pervades space and affects the people all around you.

See how even a simple apple is a continuum, a fusion of sunlight, water, earth, air, and the trees and apples that came before it. Imagine the kindness and work of the many people and creatures who have caused you to finally have this apple. Where does this apple-energy begin or end? Where does your field of energy begin or end?

Imagine your friends and companions. See them as merely a series of perceptual snapshots of a continuum of being. See the forest, flowers, objects as simply a process. Trace the fabric in your shirt back to its organic roots in the earth. See everything as interwoven pathways of light and energy unfolding through space and time. People, planets, galaxies, atomic clouds of energy, whirling, unfolding beginninglessly and endlessly through time and space. Thoughts, dreams, fantasies, and memories—all the play and process of your mind.

Exhaling, imagine releasing some old grudge or limitation. Inhaling, receive new strength, wisdom, and energy. Use your cycles of breath to let go of old limiting postures, attitudes, and emotions that keep you from moving freely through life. With each breath, receive inspiration to nurture those qualities you wish to strengthen.

Life is made of moments. What ripens in any moment are seeds sown in the past. In this moment choose consciously to sow seeds for happiness and health in the future.

Breathe your awareness into this moment.

As you exhale, allow your continuum to unfold with peace, balance, and joy.

▼▼ Nature ever flows, stands never still.
     Motion or change is her mode of existence.
     The poetic eye sees in Man the Brother of the River
     and in Woman the Sister of the River.

Their life is always transitions.
Hard blockheads only drive nails
all the time; forever...fixing.
Heroes do not fix, but flow,
bend forward ever and
invent a resource for every moment.

Ralph Waldo Emerson

4 INVESTIGATING THE MIND ▼ ▼ ▼

One should realize that one does not meditate in order to go deeply into oneself and withdraw from the world.... There should be no feeling of striving to reach some exalted or higher state, since this simply produces something conditioned and artificial that will act as an obstruction to the free flow of the mind.... When performing the meditation practice, one should develop the feeling of opening oneself out completely to the whole universe with absolute simplicity and nakedness of mind.... Meditation is not to develop trance-like states; rather it is to sharpen perceptions, to see things as they are. Meditation at this level is relating with the conflicts of our life situations, like using a stone to sharpen a knife, the situation being the stone.

Trungpa Rinpoche

Within the mind we experience a ceaseless flow of cognitive, emotional, and sensory experiences. Ordinarily our attention wanders, we are lost in our thoughts and only superficially aware of what is taking place within or around us. With mindful observation of our experience, we grow more sensitive to what we are perceiving, feeling, thinking, and doing. More in touch with ourselves, we are more in touch with the world. Old reactive patterns fall away revealing the natural power, wisdom, and love that is the mind's true nature.

The following sequence of exercises is excellent for developing insight into how your mind works. For best results, practice the first exercise for a few days or weeks, discover what insight arises, and then move on to the next until eventually you have completed the sequence.

EXERCISE 1: FOCUSING AND QUIETING THE MIND

Sit comfortably and take a few minutes to relax. Rest your hands in your lap, and quietly and gently smile to yourself. Bring your attention to your breath and feel the sensation of the air flow out of your nostrils. Now, start to count each exhalation, from one to ten. If you lose count, return to one. If you are able to reach ten, start again at one.

You can use this technique at any time during the day, even for a few minutes. The aim is to bring your attention to a keen yet relaxed focus on what you are doing. Don't try too hard to concentrate, but allow your mind to be alert and relaxed. Inevitably your mind will wander, but whenever it does simply return to the next breath. With practice you will gradually find it easier to keep your mind on whatever you are doing.

EXERCISE 2: WATCHING THE MIND

Again, sit comfortably, smile to yourself, and watch your flow of breath for a few moments. Allow the turbulence of your wandering mind to subside naturally, and allow the natural clarity and calm of your mind to become apparent.

Rest your hands palm down on your legs and bring your attention to your breath. Whenever your mind wanders off to memories or thoughts of the past, gently tap your left leg. If you notice that your mind wanders off into projected fantasies of future events, gently tap your right leg. With the mind calm yet alert, watch the breath flow, simply noting the excursion of your mind into memories and fantasies for the future. As the thoughts arise, mentally note "memory" or "fantasy," then return your attention to the breath.

The goal of this exercise is to simply notice the *process* of our thinking minds, without becoming involved in or identifying with the specific *content* of the thoughts themselves.

EXERCISE 3: SENSORY EXPERIENCE

Begin as in the previous exercises, using the breath to help you stabilize and focus your mind. Now, expand your ability to notice your mental process by including sensory experiences. Whenever you become aware of physical sensation either make the mental note "feeling" or, if you want to be more specific, "pleasure," "pain," "tingling," "itching," etc. Do not engage in internal dialogue, but simply and crisply note what you are experiencing and bring your awareness back to your breath. Likewise, when you become aware of other sensory experiences, note "hearing," "tasting," "smelling," "touching."

EXERCISE 4: EMOTIONAL FEELINGS

Begin by relaxing your body and focusing your mind with a few moments of watching the breath flow. Then, in addition to noting sensory experiences, also note your emotional experiences. Whenever a particular feeling predominates, note its nature, such as "anger," "sadness," "fear," "resentment," "guilt," "anxiety," or whatever brief mental label that fits. Pay particular attention to experiences of "liking" and "disliking." Once again, do not become involved with the content of the emotions, simply note them and return to awareness of the breath.

EXERCISE 5: INTENDING

Once we have become familiar with recognizing our thoughts and feelings as they arise, we will be able to see that prior to every voluntary action there is a mental intention. Begin now to notice this intending phase of your experience.

Mentally note the intention to stand up before getting off a chair, the intention to reach out before you open a door. Note the intention to move, to stop, to speak, to turn, to speed up or slow down, to be harsh or to be kind.

By developing mindfulness of your intention, you will develop greater power for creative choice, for seeing a whole new range of options that we hadn't seen before and that are available to us despite the habitual and highly conditioned mode that most of us live in. So, as you develop insight into the often unconscious and habitual impulses that direct your behavior, you will discover even greater freedom and power to choose both what you do and how you do it.

It is inevitable that in the fast pace of daily life you will get caught up and carried along by habitual and conditioned thoughts and emotional feelings, and that you will lose your focus of attention and the ability to consciously choose what to do or say. When you become aware of this, mentally stop, smile to yourself, and perhaps even chide yourself playfully—and then breathe and allow your thoughts and feelings to move and flow, and your sense of strength, calm, and clarity to grow.

▼▼ This is the meaning...of increasing or raising consciousness... taking functions that ran on automatic that were often incongru-ent within yourself as well as to an outside observer, and making them more conscious, more congruent, making you less the victim of automatization and more a person who understands his or her own psychological machinery and consciously controls it.

Charles Tart

5 THOUGHTS ▼ ▼ ▼

In the development of wisdom, one quality of mind above all others is the key to practice. This quality is mindfulness, attention, or self-recollection. The most direct way to understand our life situation, who we are and how our mind and body operate, is to observe with a mind that simply notices all events equally. This attitude of non-judgmental, direct observation allows all events to occur in a natural way. By keeping the attention in the present moment, we can see more and more clearly the true characteristics of our mind and body process.

Jack Kornfield

While some traditions may focus attention upon a physiological process such as breath or posture as the object of meditation, other techniques emphasize attention to the changing nature of thoughts, feelings, sensations, emotions, and states of consciousness.

Let's examine a meditation using thoughts. Though many people experience thoughts as a distraction to their meditation practice, thoughts can make an interesting and effective object of meditation. By making thoughts the object of our attention we come to the profound understanding that one is not one's thoughts. We realize that thoughts are merely bubbles floating in the vast ocean of one's mind, or simply clouds that arise, change, and pass in the sky of mind. By learning to consciously not identify with the contents of one's thoughts, one learns to view thinking as a process that will arise and unfold without the need of a "thinker." Looking deeply into our thoughts of who we are, we find that we are far more and greater than all the voices and ideas that arise and pass in the open clear space of mind.

Begin by sitting quietly and attending to the natural inflow and outflow of the breath. As thoughts arise, make a mental note of "thinking...thinking." Once recognized, many trains of thought will be derailed and the mind will once again become quiet. Practice noticing the thoughts quickly, before they have swept you off into association and elaboration. As the thoughts subside, simply return to attending to the flow of the breath. Allow thoughts to be like waves on the surface of a vast ocean, or like clouds floating in an incomprehensibly vast sky of mind.

LABELING THOUGHTS

For some people labeling the different kinds of thought processes is helpful. This can be done as follows: When memories arise in the mind, note "remembering." When fantasies of the future arise, note "imagining" or "planning." Such labeling can help to strengthen the focus and clarity of the mind and help you to identify and dissect the predominant patterns of thought that you have compulsively identified with and been impelled by throughout your life. In learning to simply recognize thinking as thinking, planning as planning, blaming as blaming, remembering as remembering, we can begin to find our power in the present moment and free ourselves from the prison of identifying with the limiting patterns of our thoughts. In this way the power of our minds can be understood and properly directed toward energizing the development of the deeper qualities of human beingness.

As you practice this meditation, guard against identifying with the content of the thoughts in the mind. Simply pay close attention to the *process* of thinking rather than the *content* of the thoughts. Pay particular attention to the compulsive and reflexive tendency to generate thoughts about your thoughts and to engage in inner commentary about the thoughts. Don't regard thoughts as good or bad, right or wrong, or as hindrances to your meditation practice. As Suzuki Roshi, a great contemporary Zen master, wrote in his book *Zen Mind Beginners Mind*:

▼▼   When you are practicing Zazen meditation, do not try to stop your
        thinking. Let it stop by itself. If something comes into your mind, let it
        come in and let it go out. It will not stay long. When you try to stop

your thinking, it means you are bothered by it. Do not be bothered by anything. It appears that the something comes from outside your mind, but actually it is only the waves of your mind and if you are not bothered by the waves, gradually they will become calmer and calmer.... Many sensations come, many thoughts and images arise but they are just waves from your own mind. Nothing comes from outside your mind.... If you leave your mind as it is, it will become calm. This mind is called Big Mind.

NOTING AND NOTICING CHANGING STATES OF MIND

As the mind becomes more stable and balanced, you may feel that the practice of labeling or noting thoughts, emotions, or phases of the breath seems cumbersome. Once you have reached this level of mental subtlety, begin to simply *notice* the inhalation or exhalation, or the type of thought or emotional state without generating a mental label. The practice of mindfully noticing the rising and passing thoughts, physical sensations, emotional feelings, and states of consciousness allows the mind to penetrate more deeply into the essential nature of these experiences.

If you find that the clarity or precision of your attention begins to fade, simply return to breath awareness or mental noting techniques in order to sharpen the focus of your attention. Once the clarity and lucidity of mind has been reestablished, let go of "noting" and return to simply "noticing" the ever changing flow of states of mind and body that are woven into the fabric of your experience.

▼▼ We asked our teacher, "What is the nature of the mind?"
He replied with the following meditation: "At your heart, imagine your mind as a drop of light which is the color of the sky and the size of a mustard seed. Imagine that this luminous drop of mind expands as far as it can. Find which is larger, the expanded drop or the sky." For fifteen minutes we sat engaged in this meditation, at which time he said, "This is the nature and expanse of the mind!"

Someone told us a story about the medicine woman, Twyla Two Wolves. She was once asked about her name and about the large necklace she wore that had two wolves heads on it. She explained that one wolf was very strong, dominating, and could be violent or vengeful at times. The other wolf was a fierce but compassionate and loving protector that nurtured and protected life. When Twyla was asked which wolf was strongest in her life, she smiled and replied, "The one I feed the most! Our minds spin many stories that we come to believe and mistake for reality. These stories manifest as images and emotionally charged thoughts that generate responses in our bodies and compel us into action. It is helpful to remember that our physiological responses to imagined events in our minds are equal in intensity to our responses to actual outer events. Especially in times such as these, when fearful images or thoughts are more common in our minds, it is very important that we learn to be mindful of and to manage the creative activity of our minds as it manifests our thoughts and emotional energies. Understanding that all acts of peace or violence begin in our minds, learning to keep the peace in our own hearts is one of the highest forms of activism.

An anthropologist once told us of an African tribe in which, from an early age, the children are trained to be mindful of their thinking. If they became aware of a foreboding or fearful thought they are instructed to counter the thought by saying to themselves, "This is a story that doesn't need to happen." If they are walking through the bush and the thought comes to mind, "Oh no, what if there is a lion hiding behind that tree waiting to eat me?" or, "What will I do if the watering hole is dry?" their inner, mental response would be, "And this is a story that doesn't need to happen!"

In a similar way, if they notice a thought arise in their mind that is a hopeful story, one that paints a picture in the mind of something that would be good to experience in actuality, the children are instructed to say to themselves, "And this is a healing story."

During unsettling times, when our minds have a tendency to run away with us, using this simple strategy can be very powerful.

When you notice fearful thoughts rising in your mind, smile gently and say to yourself, "And this is a story that doesn't need to happen." Similarly, as you notice hopeful or positive thoughts in your mind, recognize and affirm them by saying, "And this is a healing story."

Taking this technique to heart is a way of strengthening mindfulness and gaining more control of our unconscious, and often self-sabotaging, inner dialogue.

For instance, if you are on a plane, or you look up at a plane flying overhead, and you notice that you are beginning to run a crash scenario through your mind, catch yourself and say, "Whoa! This is definitely a story that doesn't need to happen." If you run similarly fearful thoughts regarding other kinds of tragedies or terrors, take action to notice and address the latency in your own mind, and to neutralize it by saying, "And this is a story that doesn't need to happen." Likewise, as you watch or think about your children, and think of them realizing the greatest potentials in their lives, or as you see the people around you and envision them coming to their humanity, wisdom, and compassion, bless and energize those thoughts and potentialities by saying, "And this is a healing story."

As you watch your thoughts, listening to the stories you are telling yourself about current reality and possible futures, take heart and be mindfully responsible for the stories you feed energy to and live by.

7 STOPPING THE WAR ▼ ▼ ▼

Since wars begin in the minds of men,
it is in the minds of men that we have to erect the ramparts of peace.

From the UNESCO Charter

One day over tea, our friend and mentor the late Paul Reps, the author of *Zen Flesh, Zen Bones*, shared the following story of his studies in the Orient. At one point Reps had traveled to Japan, with plans to visit a respected Zen master in Korea. He went to the passport office in Japan to apply for his visa and was politely informed that his request was denied due to the war that had just broken out in Korea. Reps sat down in the waiting area. He had come thousands of miles intending to study with this Korean master. He was frustrated and disappointed. What did he do? He practiced what he preached. Reaching into his bag, he mindfully pulled out his thermos and poured himself a cup of tea. With a calm and focused mind, he watched the steam rising and dissolving into the air. He smelled its fragrance, experienced its tasty bitter flavor, and enjoyed its warmth and wetness. Finishing his tea, he put his cup back on his thermos, put his thermos in his bag, and pulled out a pen and paper upon which he wrote a haiku poem. Mindfully, he walked back to the clerk behind the counter, bowed, and presented him with his poem, and his passport. The clerk read it and looked up deeply into the quiet strength in Reps' eyes. Smiling, he bowed with respect, picked up Reps' visa, and stamped it for passage to Korea. The haiku read:

▼▼   Drinking a cup of tea,
     I stop the war.

Outer wars and conflicts come from and mirror the inner conflicts in each of our hearts and minds. A first step toward peace is learning to recognize the outbreak of internal conflict and war in our own minds. This is a very powerful and profound art. During times of strife our lives depend most of all on learning to carefully observe the creative activity of our own mind as it weaves impressions and stories into beliefs that shape our attitudes and values, set our priorities, drive our communications and actions in the world.

In our work with the U.S. Army Green Berets we spent nearly six months, including a monthlong silent mindfulness meditation retreat, helping the soldiers learn to "recognize and befriend their inner enemies" and to "recognize and stop the war inside" so that they would be able to behold what was really going on with clarity, to be more mindful of their options, and to make wiser choices. Be mindful of the many moments in your day when you have the opportunity to "stop the war." In this way you too will be able to say, "walking…breathing…drinking tea…driving…I stop the war!"

▼▼   Gandhi talks about meditation being as important to the nonviolent soldier as drill practice is to the conventional soldier. Nonviolence doesn't just happen. You don't just suddenly walk into the middle of conflict and know what to do. I've discovered that the people who impress me with their nonviolent behavior in violent situations are inevitably people who have trained themselves and been involved in nonviolent strategies for a while. You can't do it in a weekend workshop…one must accept nonviolence as a form of fighting, and that's very hard for people to understand. However, compassion and joy can be as contagious as war fever.

                                                Joan Baez

The technique that follows was inspired by the insight that all of life's daily activities can be transformed into meditations, even the most mundane and ordinary activities such as washing and chopping vegetables. The key to this transformation lies in the art of paying close attention to whatever is happening in the present moment. It is not the activity that determines the quality of mental aliveness but rather the energy of mindfulness that we bring to it. We all spend much of our lives doing routine and mechanical chores. Experiment with these guidelines to see how you can transform whatever you are doing into an experience of wakefulness.

1. Begin by grounding yourself. Feel the contact between the two soles of your feet and the floor. Note the feeling of your feet touching the ground and sense that the floor beneath you connects you to the earth.
2. Knees slightly bent, feel your legs growing down into the earth. Hips, thighs, legs growing down into the earth.
3. Move your awareness next into your navel center, your center of power.
4. Now allow the upper part of your body to open and become alive. As you exhale allow your shoulders to drop. With each exhalation let your eyes be soft and your jaw be loose and soft.
5. With each exhalation come back to your body. Sense your body posture.
6. Be receptive. Allow the visual sensation of the vegetables to come to you as you chop with the knife.
7. There is nothing to do but feel the sensation of the knife in your hand. Feel its hardness. Become aware of the sensation of contact, the touch of your hand on the knife. Are you squeezing more than you need to as you chop? Soften your grip.

8. Allow the feeling of the vegetable you are holding to come to you. Note the quality of its sensations.

▼▼ Feel your feet touching the floor.
Feel your knees slightly bent.
Breathe and move from the center.
Be aware of the breath.
Let the eyes be soft.
Receive.
Stay in touch with sensations.
Attend to every moment as if it were your last.
Be soft and alert, relaxed and precise.
Experience mindfulness moving from moment to moment.

Practicing mindfulness of eating can be very revealing. There are many processes going on in the mind and body while we eat. As we bring our attention to the sequence of these processes, deep self-understanding can arise. For example,

The first step in eating is *seeing* the food.
Become mindful of seeing.
The next step is *intending* to reach for it.
Become mindful of intending.
The intention drives the body into action to *reaching* for a bite of the food.
Again become mindful of the process of moving.
When your hand or fork touches the food there is the sensation
  of touching.
Become mindful of this experience of *touching*.
Next, your arm is raised, *lifting* the food to your mouth.
Be mindful of lifting, and then of opening your mouth...of the moment
  the food touches your tongue, and of the blast of taste sensations as
  they arise, change, and fade.

Carefully notice each phase of the process. As the food comes toward your mouth notice *opening* the mouth, *putting* the food in, *lowering* the arm, *feeling* the texture of the food in the mouth, then *chewing* and *tasting*. Be particularly mindful of the experience of tasting. Notice how, as you chew, the taste disappears. Then *swallowing*. Next, watch how desire for more arises, leading to the intention to reach for another bite.

Experience how one phase seems to mechanically lead to the next as though there is really no one eating, but only a sequence of related events unfolding: intention, movement, touch sensations, tastes, and so on. Mindful eating can reveal the way in which we and our life are just a sequence of happenings, a process and flow of life energy. It can also mirror to us many of our compulsive attitudes toward consuming the universe or receiving nourishment through all of our senses. As we learn to step back and notice the process as well as the content of our activities, we can begin to recognize and transform many old and limiting patterns and choose new and more creative options for how to live our lives.

10 WALKING MEDITATION ▼ ▼ ▼

Every path, every street in the world is your walking meditation path.
Thich Nhat Hanh

Walking meditation provides a welcome method for bringing a meditative mind into action. Mindfully walking is an excellent method of meditation, especially at times when the mind is agitated and it is difficult to sit quietly.

Begin by noticing the sequence of movements as you walk...standing, lifting, moving, and placing one foot and shifting your weight...then lifting, moving, placing, and shifting your weight to the other foot. Start off slowly. Move no faster than you are able to move with complete awareness. This is not a moving meditation so much as an exercise in developing a continuity of mindful awareness. At times experiment with walking more swiftly, simply noting each time a foot touches the ground. Be loose and natural. Experience the flow of movement, moment to moment, with awareness.

Remember, the goal is not to get somewhere. Each moment that you are fully present in the flow of movement, you have arrived at your destination.

(See also *Concentration while walking* pp. 73–74.)

11 SLEEPING MEDITATION ▼ ▼ ▼

There are numerous approaches to using your sleep as a gateway to meditation. One method is to simply meditate and relax before you go to bed. You might take a few minutes to center and calm your mind. Then review the day mentally. Appreciate your day and as you notice moments about which you might feel some regret, appreciate the positive lessons that these mistakes may hold for your actions in the days to come. In your heart say "thank you" to everyone who contributed to your learning and growth today. In your heart, give and ask forgiveness where needed, and feel as though you can sleep in peace.

One technique of sleeping meditation is to imagine that your bed is within a large luminous lotus bud or a small temple or pavilion of light. Imagine that this space resonates with a healing and regenerating light that infuses you as you sleep. Imagine that the resonance and light of this space surrounds you with a buffer zone against any harsh interferences of the outer world. Imagine that it draws into itself all of the positive energy of the universe that may be helpful for you. Rest deeply, and upon awakening simply dissolve this visualization into rainbow light and absorb its essence into you.

Another method is to imagine that as you sleep you rest your head in the lap of a special teacher or protector who watches over you. Let all of your thoughts and cares be dissolved by their presence. Receive their love, strength, and inspiration as you sleep. Upon awakening, dissolve them into rainbow light and melt them into space. This technique can be combined with the previous method.

Yet another technique is to imagine as you lie in bed that with each breath you become filled with more and more light and space. As you exhale, you and everything in the universe melt into an ocean of light and space. Let your mind completely open like a drop falling into a luminous ocean. Rest deeply and powerfully. Upon awakening, let body and world appear fresh and new.

▼▼ Once upon a time,
　　I, Chuang Tzu,
　　dreamt I was a butterfly,
　　fluttering hither and thither,
　　to all intents and purposes a butterfly.
　　I was conscious only of following my fancies
　　as a butterfly,
　　and was unconscious
　　of my individuality as a man.
　　Suddenly
　　I awakened,
　　and there I lay,
　　myself again.
　　Now
　　I do not know
　　whether I was then a man
　　dreaming I was a butterfly,
　　or whether I am now
　　a butterfly dreaming
　　I am a man.
　　　　　Chuang Tzu

12 WAKING UP WITHIN THE DREAM ▼ ▼ ▼

Our truest life is when
we are in our dreams awake.
Thoreau

Many contemplative teachings describe meditation as a way to wake up within the dream of our lives. Take to heart the following wonderful insights and allow them to inspire you in this awakening.

▼▼ How do we know what reality is? When we dream at night, we believe it is reality, we feel it, we experience it. Then we wake up and discard these beliefs. How do we distinguish the real from the unreal? Where is last night's dream now? Where is yesterday's experience? You may look upon this waking state as a dream. If you see nighttime dreams and daytime illusions as the same, this can alleviate suffering. Once you establish that your experience is a dream, it may not seem so bad. Dreams are unreal, false ideas, illusions. You can see that your experience is not as serious as you thought. Your personality changes and your relationship with other people and the world is improved. There are different ways to achieve realization, but looking upon existence as a dream is one of the best, because it is very enjoyable, very satisfying and interesting. For a long time we have viewed the world in one way—as real, solid, and concrete. Seeing it differently is very enjoyable. Everything becomes easier. Nothing

is wrong: boredom is forgotten. We understand what
unity is, what infinity is—infinite time, infinite space,
infinite consciousness. When you strip away all the layers
of ideas, tensions, and frustrations, and uncover the naked
reality of consciousness—where there are not things to hold
on to—there can be nothing wrong. This is not a fantasy or
an escape. This is true. If you can realize this awareness,
the world will reveal itself as a source of unending delight.

Tarthang Tulku

▼▼ When we experience this universe we live within
as a field of reality, understand the waves and the troughs
of different dreams that weave the world we know,
then there is no longer the need to manipulate…
right relationship means right relationship with the elements,
the land, the sacred directions…. The seed of pure mind
is within all people. It is always there. It is not made impure.
Our actions may be impure and set up a stream of reactions,
but always we can come again to that seed of pure mind and
right relationship…it is time now for people to choose.
The first step is to see the power of your own consciousness….
The common kernel is care for all beings, good relationship,
cycles of reciprocity, generosity, giving of oneself, being an
empty bowl so you can know what is.

Dhyani Ywahoo

13 WAKING UP
THROUGHOUT THE DAY ▼ ▼ ▼

Our highest potential as a species is our ability to achieve full self-reflective consciousness or "knowing that we know." Through humanity's awakening, the Universe acquires the ability to look back and reflect back on itself—in wonder, awe, and appreciation.

Duane Elgin

Your meditation practice can and should begin with the first moment that you are aware that you are awake each day. This is a very important point because many people go through the large part of their day without every really being present, mindful, or fully awake. In the absence of mindfulness, habit runs our lives, and most of us get out of bed, go through our morning rituals, interact with the people in our life, drive to work, and begin our day without ever really being aware that we are awake. It may be many hours after getting out of bed before there is finally a moment of true self-reflective awareness in which you are actually mindfully aware that you are awake to a new day. However, if you train well in meditation practice, this moment may come with the first instant of awakening from sleep—before your eyes are even open—when you gently smile to yourself as you become aware of your body...aware of your thoughts... aware of your surroundings...aware that you are aware and awake.

If you like, find a physical gesture that helps you to anchor and affirm this special moment when you are first aware that you are awake to a new day. This gesture may be to reach up and touch your heart, to wiggle your toes, to mindfully bow, or to simply smile knowingly to yourself.

Awake to the blessings and opportunities of a new day, do a "systems check," and give thanks for the freedoms and faculties available to you. Send a wave of appreciation and gratitude that you can still move your body…that your eyes still see…that your ears can still hear…and that you are mentally and physically as intact and fully functioning as you are. If your faculties or senses are in any way impaired, then appreciate and rejoice in whatever capacities and faculties you do have available to you that enrich the quality of your life. Pause in this moment of awakening to be grateful for the gifts and opportunities of this fresh beginning, and this new day. Then ask yourself, "How do I want to live this day?" Knowing that the fact of death is certain, but the time of death is uncertain, reflect for a moment on the preciousness of this life and the impermanence that is the nature of each moment.

Consider the opportunities that this new day brings and the challenges of the day. What are the strengths of character or spirit that these circumstances invite you to develop and awaken more fully in yourself this day?

Give yourself the gift of a few more moments of reflective meditation now to consciously clarify the values, priorities, or principles that are most important for you to remember this day. Is today about "being present," or about "being patient," or about "deep listening," or about "being kind," or about "waking up"? Set an intention to focus on at least one spiritual quality or faculty that you would like to practice cultivating today. If it works for you, capture the essence of what you want or need to remember in a word, or short phrase that you can recall and refer back to frequently throughout the day.

Then, frequently throughout the day wake up from the momentum of the habits that lead you to live mindlessly or to not be fully present to your life. When you notice that you have been mindlessly going through the motions of your life, work, and relationships without really being there, then gently smile to yourself with compassion, and wake up…again…and again… throughout the day.

Let there be many moments of awakening throughout your busy day. If you like, in these moments, reach up again and touch your heart, wiggle your toes, or snap your fingers to physically affirm this moment of awakening. Refresh your mindfulness. Remember and recall the word or phrase that reminds you of what you hold most dear and essential to your life and success today. Then, carry this renewed clarity, focus, and commitment with you as you step fully present and awake into the next situation that your life presents. As you learn to wake up and be more present to what is going on within and around you, you will awaken to greater freedom in every realm of your life.

We are luminous being. We are perceivers. We are an awareness.
We are not objects. We have no solidity. We are boundless. The world
of objects and solidity is a way of making our passage on earth con-
venient. It is only a description that was created to help us. We, or
rather our reasons, forget that the description is only a description and
thus we entrap the totality of ourselves in a vicious circle from which
we rarely emerge in our lifetime.... We are perceivers. The world that
we perceive is an illusion. It was created by a description that was told
to us since the moment we were born.

Carlos Casteneda

We live in a world with two domains of reality. There is the domain
of conventional reality in which I am me and you are you, where
this object you hold in your hands is a book, and all objects have
names and defined relationships. Then there is the mysterious domain of
ultimate reality, the quantum soup, the implicate order, the domain of space-
time and energy that is completely empty of isolated entities and that is the
wholeness of all fields and continuums of interrelated energy and life.

Bringing an awareness of these two realities into our meditation practice
and into our daily life can help us in so many ways large and small. And life
can help us to maintain a dual perspective that embraces both a "cosmic"
view and one fully "grounded" in our present "ordinary" reality.

▼▼ There is the dual nature of self: The incomplete self and the complete
self.... As humans, we are seeing from the perspective of the incom-

plete self. This incomplete self is undoubtedly very important. But if we attach to this incomplete self, although this incomplete self is important, then we'll never be able to experience the complete self. We Zen people say, if you believe in God, this complete self means the same thing as God. That is, it shares the same standpoint as God.

Joshu Sasaki Roshi

Many disciplines of meditation function to refine and mature consciousness to such a degree that we come to two very profound discoveries regarding the nature of our "self." The first is the discovery that our ordinary identity is only "relatively real." It is a fabrication that, upon examination, is more like a creatively composed story, or historical novel, than an actual factual description of reality. The second is that there are dimensions of our selves that are universal in nature, and, as such, they extend beyond our body and beyond the duration of the life of this body. The relationship between the relative and universal dimensions of our selves is often described as being similar to the relationship between a particle, which has a relative form and location, and a field, which is nonlocalized and infinite in extension.

Such teachings are widely found in both Eastern and Western mystical traditions, and increasingly appear in contemporary cognitive science and advanced research on the nature of human consciousness. Due to a lack of discipline—or some would say a lack of grace—most people go throughout their whole life without ever awakening to the relativity of their ordinary self, or to the more universal and transcendent dimensions of themselves. Yet, when through discipline or by grace, people do awaken to these two profound realities, they are able to live their lives and face their deaths with far greater faith, confidence, compassion, and wisdom—and with much less fear.

▼▼ Emptiness is two things at once:
the absence of self and the presence of the Divine.
Thus as self decreases, the Divine increases.

Sister Bernadette Roberts

S it comfortably, cross-legged, smiling gently like a buddha, and resting easily and naturally in the flow of your breathing. Allow the breath to bring your attention to your heart center, and sense that there is a small radiant buddha of light sitting on a lotus in the center of your heart. You may see this image clearly, or just sense its potentiality there as a sphere of radiance or point of light within your heart.

When it feels natural, allow this radiant buddha and its sphere of light to grow larger and larger…until it become exactly the same size as your body. Feel yourself completely lighted up from within, suffused with this radiant enlightening energy. Rest in this contemplation.

Then, when you are ready, allow this radiant buddha that is now the size of your body to continue to expand and to grow larger and larger until you sense your body sitting like a little radiant buddha in the heart of a much larger buddha. Then envision that this larger buddha actually sits at the center of the heart of an even larger buddha who in turn sits at the heart of an even larger buddha who in turn sits within the heart of an endless cascade of radiant buddha-bodies extending to the farthest reaches of the universe—and infinitely beyond.

In a similar way, as you again envision a radiant buddha in a sphere of light at your heart-center, you may discover that sitting within its heart is, yes, another radiant buddha…and within its heart is a radiant buddha…who in turn sits within the heart of an endless fractilian cascade of radiant buddhas opening into the most minute particles and wavelengths of imagination and extending infinitesimally within.

Sitting poised within and between these infinite expanses, envision now that all of these radiant buddhas can telescope into each other bringing all into one, or expanding one into all. In the same way, envision that all beings, knowingly or unknowingly, at some essential dimension of their being, truly abide in this multidimensional universe in a similarly mysterious and miraculous way. In this way, when you "light up" a moment of mindfulness in your own mind, imagine that it resonates with and lights up that potential in the minds of all beings. When you light up a moment of love, compassion, or joy, imagine and affirm that it activates a similar potential in the hearts and minds of all beings.

▼▼ Just as a human body, though it is made up of many parts,
is a single unit because all these parts, though many, make
one body, so it is with Christ....
You all together are Christ's body.
Saint Paul

To know how to wonder and question
is the first step of the mind
toward discovery.

Louis Pasteur

Reflective meditation is a powerful form of contemplative "thinking" that is helpful for bringing a deeper wisdom and insight to your life and work. Though many people think that meditation is about stopping thoughts, such statements reflect a basic ignorance about the nature of mind and the many methods of meditation—some of which actually use disciplined thinking and analysis. In fact, we've heard the Dalai Lama say that the spiritual potency and liberating effect of reflective meditation can be far greater than the effects of meditations that merely seek to calm and quiet the mind.

To begin this meditation, sit comfortably, and focus your mind with three deep and full inhalations and exhalations.

Quietly observe the flow of breath for a few minutes, inhaling and exhaling with a relaxed yet alert quality of attention. When your mind wanders, return your attention to the breath flow.

Then, bring to mind and reflect upon a compelling question in your life, a life or work challenge or project, a verse of scripture, or an inspiring idea that you would like to be able to bring a deeper insight, wisdom, or appreciation to. In a disciplined way now, allow both your attention and your thinking to focus on this idea or theme. Reflect upon, analyze, investigate and explore its meaning, relationships, importance, and applications to your life in a deeply penetrating way.

As insights arise and culminate into a sense of *"Aha!"* shift your attention from actively reflecting on the question or theme to mindfully holding the experience or feeling of the insight. Allow that insight to soak in and to reveal its most essential understanding to your intuitive intelligence.

Then, when thoughts begin to move again in your mind, focus them back into reflecting upon the theme or question you have selected and take your investigation to a deeper level.

At the conclusion of the session take three deep, slow breaths, open your eyes, stretch your body, and if you like, record your insights. Most important, apply your insights to your daily life!

▼▼ When you eventually see through the veils
to how things really are,
You will keep saying again and again,
This is certainly not like we thought it was!
Rumi

A classic Zen approach to reflective meditation is to ask, "What is this?" When confronted with an object or a situation, rather than attempting to analyze it, simply inquire, "What is this?" and let the mind gain direct insight into it by being completely open, receptive, alert, and investigative.

▼▼ The important thing is not to stop questioning.
Albert Einstein

A related approach is to frequently remind yourself that, "I'm only labeling this as…. What is this really?" Your labeling or naming something is simply an assertion or an imputation of a concept upon a mysterious many-dimensional reality. Understand the relativity of your assertions and mental projections. Open your mind to glimpse the truly mysterious nature of things unnamed and, before thought, fresh, alive, and uncontrived.

▼▼ We live in illusion and the appearance of things.
There is a Reality.

You are that Reality.
Seeing this, you know that you are everything.
And being everything, you are no-thing.
That is all.

Kalu Rinpoche

In considering yourself, investigate and question, "Who am I?" Listen and look for answers that arise amid the ever-changing flow of physical sensations, emotional feelings, states of mind or consciousness that constellate as "your self." Within this ever changing flow of experiences, beware of any idea or assertion that you impose upon the totality of the many-dimensional mystery that is you. Experience and realize that you are far more than your thoughts of who you are…far more than you can ever imagine! Discover this reality!

▼▼   Wisdom tells me I am nothing.
Love tells me I am everything.
And between the two my life flows.

Nisargadatta Maharaj

17 STANDING IN THE POSSIBILITY ▼ ▼ ▼

Whether you believe you can or you believe
that you can't, you are right.

Henry Ford

As you begin this reflective meditation, mentally project yourself to a time five years into the future. Imagine yourself as you would most like to be, having accomplished the things you'd like to accomplish, having learned what you would like to learn, and having made the contributions you would like to have made. Now consider:

▼▼ What are the qualities you have developed in yourself?
What are the most important lessons you have learned?
What contributions do you feel most happy about having made?
In order to make these contributions, how did you have to stop underestimating yourself?
In order to make these contributions, how did you have to stop underestimating other people?
In order to make these contributions, what have you stopped pretending you cannot do?
In order to make these contributions, what strengths have you been willing to acknowledge in yourself?
In order to accomplish these things, what strengths have you learned to acknowledge in others?

Now, standing in the present moment, consider what you can do right now in order to begin to accomplish these things and make these contributions.

If it feels right, make a commitment to yourself to take this creative vision to heart and make it a living reality.

▼▼ Man has always known; he has known that life is fundamentally good, that the universe, the stars in the sky, the animals, plants, minerals, the elements of earth are not malevolent, but cosmically saturated with the purpose that gives order. The purpose is the inherent sacredness, the order of the universe itself. As long as man has kept this sacredness before him, indeed, as long as he has woven it into the pattern of his heart through humility and spiritual attunement, the pattern of human society has also reflected the sacredness and order with which all things are endowed.

Jose Arguelles

18 MEDITATION
ON THE FIVE ELEMENTS ▼ ▼ ▼

Begin this meditation with a few minutes of relaxation and breath awareness. Now bring your attention to the earth element of your body—that aspect of your existence which is dense and solid. Feel the massiveness of your body, its weight and form. As you breathe, contemplate and feel the element of earth experienced as form, density, mass, and weight.

Now shift your focus of attention to the water element—that aspect of your body and of your world which is fluid and cohesive. Feel or imagine this dynamic fluidity as blood, lymph, and other waters of life flowing within your body. Sense and imagine this water element flowing through the world in which you live.

Next, attend to the fire element. The element of fire is associated with the warmth, light, and heat of your body, and of the world. Feel this inner heat, this vital warmth that dissipates at death. Experience how this element of heat and light is evident as it radiates in all living beings and through the world around you.

Now bring your attention to the air element. The air element is related to the spaces of the internal cavities, movement, and the flow of the breath. This function of respiration dynamically connects you to your world. At a more subtle level, this air element is associated with the movement of subtle energies throughout the subtle energy systems of the body sometimes pictured in acupuncture or esoteric anatomy charts. On a macro scale, this element weaves the web of resonant energies that regulate the metabolism of the planet, and entrain and attune us with the movements of the heavens. Contemplate the pervasiveness of this air/wind element within and around you.

Finally, bring your attention to the fifth element. The faculty of aware-ness or knowingness is often associated with this most essential, most sub-tle element. This element is not physical in nature. It is called by many names: consciousness, ether, mind, spirit, space, or that which does not die. This is the animating force unique to life, the vital essence that sees through our eyes, listens through our ears, and is ever awake in the heart of all liv-ing beings.

The contemplation of these five elements is used in many traditions as a means of enabling individuals to better align themselves with the inner and outer elements of life and the cosmos.

▼▼   We are part of the earth and it is part of us... The perfumed flowers are our sisters; the deer, the horse, the great eagle, these are our broth-ers. The rocky crests, the juices of the meadows, the body heat of the pony, and human beings all belong to the same family.... The shining water that moves in the streams and rivers is not just water but the blood of our ancestors.... The rivers are our brothers, they quench our thirst.... The air is previous to the red man, for all things share the same breath—the beast, the tree, the man, they all share the same breath.... The air shares its spirit with all the life it supports. The wind that gave our grandfather his first breath also receives his last sigh.... What are human being without the beasts? If all the beasts were gone, human beings would die from a great loneliness of spirit, for whatever happens to the beasts soon happens to all human beings. All things are connected. This we know. The earth does not belong to man; man belongs to the earth. This we know. All things are connected like the blood which unites one family. All things are connected. Whatever befalls the earth befalls the children of the earth. Man does not weave the web of life, he is merely a strand in it. Whatever he does to the web, he does to himself.

Chief Seattle

19 HOLLOW BODY MEDITATION ▼ ▼ ▼

Wealth, position, and power become tiresome if the spiritual nature is not satisfied in its quest for meaning. As life progresses, the value of meditation and the cultivation of qualities of joy, equanimity, compassion, and love which give life its nobility and value will become more important. Amidst gain and loss, fame and defame, praise and blame, happiness/pleasure and sorrow/pain, the Awakened One urged us to keep a balanced mind. Only in this state can deep understanding arise, and the heart attain peace.

Rina Sircar

One of the most effective techniques for dissipating accumulated stress and tension is to experience your body as hollow—open and filled with clear space. Experience this space as neither solid nor empty, but rather as an inner openness within which feelings and sensations can freely come and go. This inner openness and spaciousness is devoid of any obstruction or any sense of solidity and denseness.

This deceptively simple method has been used for thousands of years and has recently been extensively documented to promote the integration and optimization of neuromuscular, autonomic, and central nervous system functions, as well as to reduce pain and enhance endurance and overall mindbody integration.

Begin by sitting comfortably with your spine straight and your body relaxed.

Now, bring your attention to the breath, and as you inhale imagine drawing your attention into your head. It may be helpful to imagine the breath like a luminous crystal mist that completely fills your head. As you breathe out, let go of the image or feeling of denseness or solidity and imagine this region as completely open and filled with space. Sense and feel the sensations and vibrations that come and flow freely within this open space inside your head.

As you next breathe in, draw your attention into your neck and throat, and again as you breathe out, imagine this region is left filled with space— a space open to the flow of life energy, vibration, and sensation. Experience a sense of inner openness, a space free from denseness or solidity.

Continue now to breathe your awareness region by region into each part of your body. One region at a time, breathe this sense of luminous open space into your hands, arms, and shoulders, your chest, abdomen, hips and buttocks and genitals, and finally your legs and feet. As you exhale, feel and vividly imagine that each region is left feeling utterly open to the flowing streams of sensation and vibration that knit the fabric of your experience. Amid this flow of vibration and sensation, experience the inner quiet stillness and peacefulness that accommodate these myriad changes and vibrations.

Now simply rest in this experience of your hollow body without conceptualization or analysis. Simply allow thoughts, feelings, perceptions, and images to arise and dissolve like luminous bubbles and streams flowing within this inner space of awareness. Experience your body as unified and whole, completely open to equalizing and diffusing the accumulated pressures of your body and mind. Allow each breath to deepen this inner harmony and to energize the calm intensity of your awareness.

Initially you may find that some regions feel dense, solid, and impregnable. You may be unable to get a clear feeling for these regions. Many people have cut themselves off from parts of their body due to past injuries, surgery, abuse as a child, or other conscious or suppressed trauma. So long as there are parts of your body cut off from your sense of wholeness, parts of your brain and mind potentials are blocked as well. These "locked closets" of your body leave you vulnerable as they are often the breeding ground for degenerative disease and cancer. In this case, combine your practice of this technique with the *Mental massage* (p. 142).

Gradually and with practice you will easily be able to imagine and actually feel that your whole body, from the top of your head to the tip of your toes is completely open, unobstructed, unified, and radiant. This inner sense of your wholeness will enable you to reclaim those lost regions of your body, brain, and mind. Eventually you will be able to access this unified, open, and luminous sense of your entire body with a single breath.

ADVANCED VARIATIONS

The following variations on the hollow body technique will further enhance your mindbody coordination and self-healing abilities.

1. *Modulating body size.* Having dissolved your whole body into a unified sphere of empty openness, imagine your body in different sizes. Gradually allow your sense of your body to grow smaller and smaller. Reduce it to the size of a sesame seed and then expand it until it contains the room, the building, the globe, the Milky Way and the universe. Take as much time as you need to vividly sense and flex these undeveloped capacities of your mind. Alternate between tiny and vast as you feel comfortable, maintaining a feeling of hollowness and luminous openness throughout. Having become familiar with this technique, proceed to the following variation.

2. *Dissolving and absorbing.* Allow your body to appear and feel hollow and radiant. Then expand your awareness to fill the universe. Next, gradually imagine the entire universe dissolving down to absorb into your body. Then imagine your body dissolving from top and bottom into a small sphere of light at the center of your chest. Imagine this tiny luminous sphere growing smaller and smaller until your mind simply dissolves into a lucid empty openness.

Now rest in this empty open space: still, quiet, clear, and nonconceptual. As the first thought arises in this stillness of your mind, immediately generate yourself as your hollow body again, yet this time feel as though all of your old limiting thoughts, negative habits of perception and behavior, and physical congestions have completely dissolved into space and that you are arising fresh, clean, clear, radiant, and purified—in a sense reborn.

With frequent practice of these techniques the strength of old limiting patterns will gradually diminish, allowing you to access more effective and creative responses to the opportunities and challenges of your life.

CARRY-OVER PRACTICE

As you move through your day, carry this inner sense of unified openness and wholeness with you. Frequently use the breath to help you renew this sense. To deepen and enhance the benefits of this technique, train your mind to pay attention to the space and distance between things, and to imagine and sense the volume and natural radiance of other people and objects. Notice how the spaces between buildings, cars, people, and clouds actually connect everything. Train your inner and outer perception to experience how space, within and without, connects everything. With practice you will gradually come to attend to space and emptiness in relation to objects and things. You will learn to recognize space as a unifying medium rich in information of many frequencies and wavelengths transduced by our ordinary and subtle senses. This quality of sensitivity can further be enhanced by practicing listening for the silences between sounds and noticing the space between thoughts. This is a necessary foundation for enhancing intuition and expanding the range of your subtle senses.

This meditation will help you massage the inside of your body with your mind. Sweep your attention through your body like a gentle breeze that moves from the inside out. Allow the mind to move deeply and unobstructed throughout the body, as though everything inside you were openness and patterns of energy and space. Allow the attention to move particularly through regions of discomfort or disease. Gently direct the mind to sweep back and forth, up and down, moving like a laser beam or a floodlight, sweeping from different directions, front to back, top to bottom, diagonally or in spirals. Intuitively feel how you can best move your attention into a region of internal space, and try different approaches.

Pay particular attention to how these subtle sensations change, how everything inside you is moving, vibrating, changing moment to moment. If you have difficulty focusing your attention in this way, bring your attention to your breathing for a while, and when your concentration has been energized, return to this sweeping of mind through body.

Though at first you may work at the level of imagination, you can quickly develop the subtle, deep awareness that is able to sense, feel, and actually alter patterns of subtle sensation consciously. Though at first the body may seem riddled with discomfort, or some regions may be impossible to sense or feel at all, gradually these parts of yourself will come alive with sensation and a feeling of more harmonious resonance.

21 THE CENTER OF YOUR MANDALA ▼ ▼ ▼

In every system of sacred art and science we find reference to methods of generating a sphere of sacred space. These spheres are often represented as mandalas, medicine wheels, gothic windows, neolithic stone circles, and other sacred symbols. Each has a center and a periphery. Each serves as a tool for contemplation guiding the mind to recognize and participate more fully in the dynamic interplay of forces within and around us.

Sitting comfortably and at ease, breathe and draw the universe into you. Breathing out from the nucleus of your inner mandala, feel yourself sitting at the center of your universe. Imagine your sphere of energy and awareness opening to enfold and infuse the space around you.

Allow the flow of the breath to effortlessly remind you of your dynamic relationship with the universe. Remember that you are always at the center of your world, wherever you go. And remember that every single being likewise abides at the center of their own mandala. Interpenetrating spheres of energy and consciousness fill space with an intricate lattice work of mandalas generated from the nucleus of each atom and each being.

Each being embracing and embraced by all others.

Sit firm, confident, and serene at the center of your mandala of energy and awareness.

And if any experience knocks you off center, simply breathe and draw yourself back to the center.

Quietly and comfortably, allow the breath to freely come and flow, effortlessly releasing and dissolving thoughts and tensions into space.

As you inhale, imagine a bubble of light energy filling you from within. As you exhale, imagine this bubble expanding...opening and expanding out into the space around you. With each breath, be filled by this luminous energy, and with each exhalation, imagine this sphere of light energy opening and expanding, moving freely through the space, the walls, the buildings, the earth around you. Let everything open. Let your small sense of self expand and open to your surroundings. Allow all of the feelings and sensations and vibrations within your body to expand, open, and dissolve like a cloud melting into space. Use the breath to help you learn to expand your sphere of energy awareness like the expanding circle of a pebble dropped onto a still pool...ahhh...opening...opening...in all directions...filling the space above you, filling the space below you, expanding and opening out before you, behind you opening and expanding as a sphere of energy-life-awareness all around you...opening and expanding with each breath.

Now as you inhale, allow this light energy to take on a pleasing color and feeling quality—perhaps blue and peaceful, or red and warm, or any color-feeling combination that feels right to you. Allow this feeling and color to fill you deeply, and then as you exhale, allow the color-feeling sphere to open and expand within and around you. Imagine filling the space around you with luminous waves of warmth and well-being. Imagine generating an atmosphere of peace, of happiness and good vibrations that pervades the world around you. Sitting quietly, simply allow this wellspring of inner energy to come alive, open, and expand around you so that anyone near you can receive the benefit.

Now, having established this expansive sense of well-being, imagine that as your sphere of energy awareness opens and expands, there is an echo from the universe at large. Imagine that as your drop or nucleus of energy expands outward, a vast ocean of peace, of warmth, and of love converges and pours into you. Simultaneously, experience this feeling of expansion and convergence—your tiny mind-drop opening outward, and dissolving into a vast spacious ocean, and this ocean of positive energy vibration flowing and converging into your drop. Allow all of your limitations, pains, thoughts, and cares to be dissolved into this free-flowing convergence.

VARIATION

This is an excellent technique for dissolving emotional pain as well. As you exhale, allow the energy or feeling of the pain to open out and dissolve into space. As the energy vibration of the pain expands, sense or vividly imagine feeling a healing echo of energy vibration pouring into you from the ocean of energy surrounding you. Feel this healing wave flowing into you and dissolving into the region of the pain. For example, when you experience a sense of burning, allow that feeling to expand while simultaneously a cool, soothing energy is drawn back into you. If you are feeling agitated, allow that feeling to open, expand, and dissipate while at the same time you feel deep peace pouring into you, flooding you completely with well-being. Allow yourself to receive from the universe-at-large whatever you most need at this time.

Breathing out, give yourself permission to let go of the knots of tension that block your body, fog your mind, and block your heart. Let everything within you open into harmony. Allow the breath to naturally and effortlessly bathe your tissues in oxygen and light that dissolve the tensions or pains. Allow the waves of breath to fill you with the love, the courage, and the strength that you need to let go of tension, to let go of fear, to release doubt or anger, and to rest in your own wholeness.

▼▼ Breathing and receiving what you need...
releasing the old limitations...
resting in wholeness...
tune into whatever frequency of positive healing qualities you need
at this time.

23 TRANSFORMING EMOTIONS ▼ ▼ ▼

The mystics ask you to take nothing on mere belief. Rather, they give you a set of experiments to test in your own awareness and experience. The laboratory is your own mind, the experiment is meditation.

Ken Wilber

Ordinarily our emotional responses are highly conditioned and automatic. Blown by the winds of our emotions, we often experience confusion, disharmony, and physical disease. Once you understand this process, you can assume more control and responsibility for how you use your emotions. You can learn to regain your balance and bring harmony to your mindbody by generating appropriate emotions as an antidote to the self-centered and often destructive aspects of your emotional reactions.

In order to work on transforming our emotional reactions, it is necessary to first understand how emotions work. One way to approach this is with the following model.

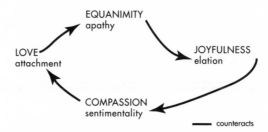

Here we have four basic emotional states followed by their potentially dark side. Each of these eight basic emotions are interrelated. In each, the emotional feeling shown in capital letters is the more matured state, expressing the true and natural human being. The emotional feeling that is indicated in small letters is the condition that you may slip into if the experience becomes tinged with self-centeredness. One is the manifestation of the true and free spark of human intelligence and the other is the self-centered, egoistic aspect that it can easily become:

Equanimity can turn to apathy,
Joyfulness to elation,
Compassion to sentimentality,
Love to attachment.

Meditation training helps you focus your attention to understand the interplay of mental attitudes, emotional feelings, and physical reactions. As you come to understand this complex process, you can maintain or restore your internal balance by generating an emotion that is an appropriate antidote to a disturbing emotional state. For instance:

Love counteracts apathy,
Equanimity will ground you from experiencing elation,
Joyfulness will melt your fixation on sentimentality,
Compassion will inhibit attachment.

If you are bored, let yourself love others who may need to feel loved. If your compassion is dissipated into sentimentality, rejoice a little, and if you become too elated, generate more equanimity to calm down.

Remember, each of our emotions can be expressed from the true essence of the human spirit or from a distorted bias of our own self-centeredness. One will set you free, while the other will perpetually entrap you in a cycle of disharmony.

OTHER STRATEGIES FOR TRANSFORMING EMOTIONS INCLUDE

1. *Take responsibility.* In an emotionally charged situation, focus your attention on the physical sensations in your body and on your own emotional feelings—not on the situation or on those involved. If you feel tension, holding, or squeezing in your body, bring your attention to those feelings. Breathe...and relax. Remember, you are the only one responsible for your mental, emotional, and physical response to the situation. Breathe, relax, and open your field of attention to find a creative solution or response to the challenge.

2. *Investigate sensations.* Investigate the physical sensations and mental images related to your emotional state. Reflect, "What does this fear, anger, sadness, or grief really feel like? Where do I feel it in my body? How big is it? Where does it come from or go to? What are the thoughts and mental tape loops associated with this emotional state?" You will find that by simply investigating the nature of your emotional reactions, the intensity will diminish. You will be able to calm and clear your mind and to respond from a state of centered strength.

3. *Open to pain.* When you feel overwhelmed by other people's pain, let that pain tear your heart open. Awaken genuine compassion: compassion for the difficulties and suffering or helplessness; compassion for your own frustration or helplessness; compassion for all others who might feel as they or you feel in that situation.

4. *Remember the cause of cruelty.* When others act cruelly or insensitively, remember that no one can act that way unless they are suffering themselves. The more quickly you are able to recognize and transform your own negative emotional patterns, the less likely you are to hurt someone else.

5. *Don't make more trouble for yourself.* Think about the irony of being angry about feeling angry, or guilty about feeling guilty. Learning to recognize and accept old conditioned emotional reactions is the first step to changing them.

6. *Befriend your emotions.* Learn to befriend your confused or negative emotions. When a negative emotion arises, smile to yourself and mentally note, "Ah, anger (or blame, guilt, or jealousy)...of course!"

7. *Develop a flexibility of emotional response.* In the face of anger, for example, practice generating compassion toward yourself and others. In the face of greed, practice generating gratitude for all that you have. Experiencing jealousy, try finding the feeling of rejoicing in the good fortune of another. When impatient, practice patience.

8. *Keep on learning.* When all else fails, learn from your experience! Analyze the situation after it's over, clarify how you might improve your response in the future, and vividly imagine yourself in a similar situation responding the way that you would like to.

As you develop the ability to authentically recognize and acknowledge what you are feeling, you will be better able to understand the destructive potential of negative emotional states. This direct understanding will enable you to consciously cultivate new and more effective emotional responses that bring greater balance and harmony to your mindbody, your behavior and relationships.

When we begin just to try to accept ourselves, the ancient
burden of self-importance lightens up considerably. Finally
there's room for genuine inquisitiveness, and we find we
have an appetite for what's out there.

Pema Chödron

As we develop in our practice of meditation we naturally become more
conscious of what is going on in our own minds. We become
clearer about what we feel and why. We start to uncover the dis-
crepancies in our lives and get in touch with the bruises and hurts of old relationships. Slowly, we are able to tie loose ends and heal the wounds.

The practice of a forgiveness meditation is a wonderful way to heal the
pain of the old hurts that block our hearts and prevent us from trusting and
loving ourselves and others. Forgiveness is the key to opening our hearts, to
learning from the painful lessons of the past in order to move into the future
unhindered.

Begin by sitting quietly, relaxing your body, and focusing your mind with
the breath. Allow memories and images and emotions to float freely in your
mind—things you have done, said, and thought that you have not forgiven
yourself for, no matter how painful they are.

From your heart, say to yourself, "I forgive myself for whatever I have
done in the past, intentionally or unintentionally, my actions, my words,
and my thoughts. I have suffered enough! I have learned and grown and I
am ready now to open my heart to myself. May I be happy, may I be free
from confusion, may I know the joy of truly understanding myself, others,

and the world. May I come to know my own wholeness and fullness and help others to do the same."

Now, in the space in front of you, imagine a person you love whom you want to forgive or whose forgiveness you need. From your heart to theirs directly communicate the following: "With all my heart I forgive you for whatever you may have done, intentionally or unintentionally, by your actions, your words or thoughts that have caused me pain. I forgive you, and I ask that you forgive me for whatever I have done, intentionally or unintentionally to you, by my actions, my words or my thoughts. I ask your forgiveness. May you be happy, free, and joyful. May we both open our hearts and minds to meet in love and understanding as we grow into wholeness." Imagine that this message is received and accepted, and affirm the feeling of healing between you. Then let the image melt into space.

Now, in the space in front of you, imagine someone toward whom you feel great resentment or negativity. To the best of your ability and from your heart to theirs, communicate the essence of the following: "From my heart I forgive you for whatever you have done, intentionally or unintentionally, that has caused me pain. I forgive you for the actions and words and thoughts that you have expressed from your own pain, confusion, insensitivity, and fear of me. I forgive you, and I ask that you forgive me for the way in which I have intentionally or unintentionally closed my heart to you. I ask your forgiveness for causing you suffering. May you be happy. May you be free from suffering and confusion. May we both open our hearts to meet in love and understanding as we grow into our wholeness." Imagine that this message has been received and accepted, and affirm the healing that has taken place within you and between the two of you. Then allow the image to melt into space.

Next, think about the countless people toward whom you have closed your heart. Remember how you felt and what you did when people abused you, spoke harshly, took "your" parking place, crowded in front of you in line, ad infinitum.... Consider how many people you have hurt in some way, by your own conscious or unconscious actions, words, and thoughts. How many times have you been the abuser, the one who crowded in, the one who spoke harshly? Imagine these countless beings standing before you. From your heart to theirs generate the essence of the following: "I forgive you for whatever you have done, intentionally or unintentionally, that has caused me to suffer. I forgive you and ask you to forgive me for whatever I have done, intentionally or unintentionally, that has hurt you. May you and I and all of us create the causes for happiness in our lives. May we outgrow and transform the causes of our suffering. May we all come to know the joy of truly understanding and experiencing our interrelationship. May we open our hearts and minds to each other and meet in harmony."

Repeat this reflective meditation as often as you like. At the conclusion, imagine and feel as vividly and wholeheartedly as you are able that you have actually released all guilt and blame toward yourself. In this present moment, allow yourself to feel forgiveness and a patient acceptance of your past actions.

25 INCREASING COMPASSION ▼ ▼ ▼

The Great Way is not difficult for those who have no preferences. When love and hate are both absent everything becomes clear and undisguised. Make the smallest distinction however and heaven and earth are set infinitely apart. If you wish to see the truth then hold no opinions for or against anything. To set up what you like against what you dislike is the disease of the mind. When the deep meaning of things is not understood the mind's essential peace is disturbed to no avail.

Sengtsan, third Zen patriarch

The following meditation is taken from a talk given by the Dalai Lama. "Avoid harming others and whenever possible be of service." If you wish to increase your compassion, you can think in this way: First, visualize yourself as a neutral person, neither particularly good nor particularly bad. Now, on the right side, visualize your old self as a person who is only ever seeking his or her own welfare, who doesn't think at all about other people, who would take advantage of anyone at any time whenever the chance arises, and who is never content. And, on the left side of your neutral self, visualize a group of people who are really suffering and need help.

Now think: All humans have the natural desire to be happy and to avoid suffering; All humans equally have the right to be happy and to get rid of suffering. Then think in a wise, not selfish way: Everybody wants happiness; nobody wants to be foolish or to be like that selfish person.

So you see, if we want to be a good person, a more reasonable, logical person, then we don't want to be like the narrow-minded selfish person on the right. We wouldn't want to join this single, selfish, greedy, discontented person on the right. If we were to draw a line between the single selfish person and the group, you would want to join the group.

When we practice this technique of visualization, naturally the majority side wins our heart. The closer you come to taking the side of the majority, the further you become from your selfishness. Because you yourself are the meditator, your own sense of altruism will increase and increase. If you practice this way daily, it will be helpful.

▼▼ The hardest state to be in is one in which you keep your heart open to the suffering that exists around you, and simultaneously keep your discriminative wisdom. It's far easier to do one or the other; to keep your heart open and get lost in pity, empathetic suffering, righteous indignation, etc.; or remain remotely detached as a witness to it all. Once you understand that true compassion is the blending of the open heart and the quiet mind, it is still difficult to find the balance. Most often we start out doing these things sequentially. We open our hearts and get lost in the melodramas, then we meditate and regain our quiet center by pulling back in from so much openness. Then we once again open and get sucked back into the dance. So it goes cycle after cycle. It takes a good while to get the balance. For at first the discriminative awareness part of the cycle makes you feel rather like a cold fish. You feel as if you have lost your tenderness and caring. And yet each time you open again to the tender emotions, you get lost in the drama and see your predicament: if you really want to help others who are suffering, you just have to develop the balance between heart and mind such that you remain soft and flowing yet simultaneously clear and spacious. You have to stay right on the edge of that balance. It seems impossible, but you do it. At first, when you achieve this balance, it is self-consciously maintained.

Ultimately, however, you merely become the statement of the amalgam of the open heart and quiet mind. Then there is no more struggle; it's just the way you are.

Ram Dass

Some day, after we have mastered the winds,
the waves, the tides, and gravity,
we shall harness the energies of love.
Then, for the second time in the history of the world,
man will have discovered fire.

Teilhard de Chardin

In this heart-centered meditation practice we focus initially upon cultivating the quality of loving-kindness for ourselves, and then gradually develop our capacity to expand the radiance of love to encompass all living beings without exception.

Begin now by affirming and recognizing that at the very core of your being dwells an essential purity of being whose radiant presence is of the nature of loving-kindness and compassion. No matter how disturbed or confused your ordinary mind may be, at this dimension of your being you touch a state of purity, infinite clarity, and compassion. There is a potential here that is fathomless, a potential for wisdom and compassion, and our very wish for well-being and happiness, our very wish to be free of suffering, may be regarded as an expression of that true nature. Let this deep, pure, and true nature of your self be unveiled, and allow it to manifest its full potential.

From this quality of sacred self-regard, allow any of your shortcomings that come to mind to awaken a natural feeling of spontaneous compassion toward yourself. With this compassion and loving-kindness, acknowledge and embrace those shortcomings and self-sabotaging attitudes or habits, and cultivate this prayer, aspiration, or wish:

▼▼ May I be free of these distortions, free of anger, free of grasping,
free of confusion, free of arrogance.

May I be free from any negative attitudes and confusions that distort
my pure and clear mind.

May I recognize and cultivate the qualities of mindful presence, of
loving-kindness and compassion, of wisdom and patience.

May I awaken and bring forth within myself all the most wholesome
and noble qualities of being that are latent within me.

For my own well-being, and for the well-being of others, may all
these qualities flourish in my life, and may they inspire others.

May I come to live in a way that nurtures a profound sense of aliveness and well-being in my life.

May I feel comfortable and at ease in my body and in my mind,
and with those I live and work with.

May I find peace, joy, and happiness within me and may I radiate
those qualities in a compassionate way, and walk on the earth with
a deeper wisdom and kindness than I have ever known.

May my anxieties, fears, and sorrows melt away and leave my
heart open, clear, radiant, and happy.

May I come to live and walk in this world in a truly balanced way,
and know the centeredness, joy, and wisdom that come from being
truly present within myself and in whatever circumstances I may find
myself.

Mentally or physically reach up and touch your heart and affirm the
awakening of these wishes in your life right now.

Now, bring to mind a loved one, a person whom you admire, respect, or
feel tenderly toward. Let this be someone toward whom it is easy and natural to feel appreciation and affection, someone whom you are always happy
to see. Reflect that this person, just like yourself, gets caught in his or her
own confusions and delusions. And just like you, this person also has incredible potential and is endowed with the true nature and deep purity of spirit.
She or he too has the potential to truly be a source of blessings to the world
and a source of inspiration for all she or he meets. Letting your heart open
toward this person, realize that she or he too yearns to live in comfort,
peace, and well-being. From your heart radiate the wish:

▼▼   May you, dear friend, like me, become ever more free from
anxiety, confusion, or negativity.
May you be free from suffering and pain.
May you awaken within yourself all the most wholesome
and life-affirming qualities of being, and may you nurture and
cultivate them so that they will grow ever stronger in your life.
May you find a path in life true to your spirit, on which you
find health, peace, and freedom, and awaken to your greatest
potentials.

Focus now on someone you simply feel neutrally toward. It might be a
grocery clerk you see frequently, a person at a gas station, a colleague, or a
person you work with for whom you have no special feeling at all. Recognize that this person too, like you, is endowed with incredible potentials,
and like you wishes to be free from the limitations, stuck places, and sufferings in his or her life. Realize and experience that this person's experience
of suffering and joy is no less real, and no less important than your own.
Though this person may have no conscious contemplative or spiritual orientation at all, still at the most fundamental level she or he yearns to be
whole, and there is within him or her a mysterious and precious quality of
presence that is universal in its nature and dimensions. Open your heart-
mind toward this person and extend your loving-kindness to him or her,
wishing:

▼▼   May you be free from pain and suffering.
May you cultivate the confidence, vitality, peace, and clarity of mind
you need to transform all confusion and negativity, and awaken
wholeheartedly to your true nature and potentials.
May you be well and happy, free of unnecessary pain, grief,
and fear.

And affirm and imagine it to be so.

Next, bring to mind someone that you really don't like, a person whom
you'd just rather not see at all, or even hear about. Perhaps it is simply certain personality characteristics in this person that irritate you. Or, perhaps
this person has wronged or hurt you in some way. Steady your self, bring

him or her to mind, and consider how this person too, just like you, wishes for happiness and to avoid the pains and sorrows of life. Maybe her or his ways of pursuing this are confused, but the wish is no less real, the experience of joy and sorrow no less real. Yet, if this person were to find effective means for taming his/her mind, opening the heart, and being more sensitive to the people around him or her, the very reasons for which you dislike that person would vanish, and a wonderful person could emerge instead.

Consider how, as with yourself, when this person's actions are driven by confusion, delusion, or by their own wounding and mental distortions, their efforts to find happiness are so unskillful that they create more suffering and harm for themselves, and for others around them. Just imagine how different things would be if they were to come to a radical healing of their wounds, if they were to balance all the turbulent and distorted mind states and energies whirling within them. Imagine how different they would be if through the power of your loving-kindness and prayers, or through their own good grace or karma, they were to awaken right now to their wholeness and to their true nature and full potentials.

With this perspective, let your heart begin to open to this person—and to all others like them—to wish them well, and to include them in the radiance of your loving-kindness:

▼▼ Just as I wish happiness for myself, may you be well and happy.
May all your afflictions fall away.
May your real beauty and highest potentials for kindness be swiftly realized, and may your True Nature be unveiled.

Imagine this to be so.

As we bring this meditation to a close, also allow this quality of loving awareness to express itself pictorially by imagining a pearl of radiant white light. This radiant pearl is of the nature of purity and the nature of loving-kindness, which is the very essence of one's own True Nature. Imagine this pearl of radiant, brilliant white light at your heart, and from an inexhaustible source, allow that light to suffuse every cell of your body, thoroughly illuminating and filling your entire body with this light of loving-kindness, of purity and purification.

Then envision your body being so filled that it is no longer able to contain this light. Rays of light reach out in all directions, in front of you and behind you, to your left and to your right, upward into the heavens and downward into the earth—infinitely expanding in all directions. As the radiance of your loving-kindness reaches forth and flows in all directions, let it carry the energy and inspiration of your loving-kindness, of your loving concern for all beings, who, like yourself, aspire for happiness and yearn to be free from suffering. Imagine these rays of light touching all the people and living beings around you—reaching out first to those in the room with you...then to those in your neighborhood...your city...your part of the country...and to the whole world.

Envision this radiance of your innermost being bringing well-being to all beings, turning into food for those who are hungry or starving...into rain where there is drought...harmony where there is conflict...peace where there is hatred or war. Let this light expand to embrace all beings on this precious planet, and let it reach out as a source of blessings and inspiration to all beings in all worlds.

In this way, dedicate the spiritual power of this meditation practice, not just to your own individual well-being, but also to the well-being, peace and awakening of the entire world and to all beings without exception.

If you close your meditation sessions at least once a day with this practice, it will add a more universal dimension to your whole practice.

▼▼ May I become at all times, both now and forever,
    A protector for those without protection,
    A guide for those who have lost their way,
    A ship for those with oceans to cross,
    A bridge for those with rivers to cross,
    A sanctuary for those in danger,
    A lamp for those without light,
    A place of refuge for those who lack shelter,
    And a servant to all in need.
                      Shantideva

The following simple version of loving-kindness meditation is easy to remember and can be used to open your heart when done as a sitting meditation practice, or as you move about through the world. Here's how it goes:

Bring your attention to your heart now and allow your breath to come and flow easily and naturally. As you repeat the following phrases quietly or silently to yourself, go for the feeling behind these words:

▼▼ May I be happy and peaceful...
    May I be free from fear...or pain...
    May I live with love and compassion...
    May I fully awaken (to my True Nature and Potentials) and be free.

Going deeper and deeper into the feeling behind the words, continue reciting this blessing of loving-kindness to yourself for as long as you like.

Then if you like, bring the radiance of this heartfelt feeling to the next step—imagining that you are opening your heart to share this deep, loving energy with a friend. From your heart, to and through his heart, extend the feeling within these phrases:

▼▼ May you be happy and peaceful...
    May you be free from fear...or pain...
    May you live comfortably and openheartedly with love and compassion...
    May you fully awaken and be free.

Open your heart to share this wave of love and blessings with your loved one or friend—or with many loved ones or friends, one at a time or as a group. Continue radiating the flow of this deep and loving feeling for as long as you like.

And now, if you like, open your heart and mind even more deeply and completely to an even more sublime level of loving-kindness. Repeating the following phrases from your heart to and through an ever expanding circle of "all your relations," expand this wave of loving-kindness to embrace all beings—those whom you know, and those unknown to you...those near and close to you, and those who are far or distant from you...those whom you love...and those who challenge you to love more deeply.
Open your heart and extend this wish to them all:

▼▼ May all beings be happy and peaceful...

May all beings be free from fear or pain...
May all beings live with love and compassion....
May all beings fully awaken and be free.

As you continue to deepen into this radiant state of loving-kindness, imagine countless beings joining in with you...as though they too are repeating these heartfelt phrases with you...extending their loving thoughts and blessings to you and to all beings everywhere:

▼▼ May all beings be happy and peaceful...
May all beings be free from fear or pain...
May all beings live with love and compassion...
May all beings fully awaken and be free.

27 DRIVING MEDITATION ▼ ▼ ▼

We received the following advice from the Venerable Gen Lam Rimpa some months before we entered a year-long silent contemplative retreat. We had gone to visit Gen-la shortly after he arrived from Dharamsala where he had been in contemplative retreat for nearly seventeen years. At the request of the Dalai Lama—who was both his mentor and colleague—Gen-la had left his retreat hut in the Himalayas and traveled to Seattle where he would train and lead about fifteen Western students in this special meditation retreat. We both very much hoped to participate in this retreat, and we realized that many things could potentially arise in our lives that would interfere with our participation. We asked Gen-la if he had any advice or meditations for averting any obstacles that might arise—problems with our parents' health, logistical glitches in being gone for a whole year, potentials for problems with our own health, juggling our finances to be on sabbatical for a whole year, and so forth. With tremendous tenderness and warmth, Gen-la offered us the following advice:

▼▼ "When you are driving down the freeway in your car, look out and see all the other people driving in cars around you rushing to reach their destinations. As you drive, open your heart to these people who, just like you, yearn for happiness and hope to avoid the sorrows of life. Reach out to these people with the wish or the prayer, 'May you safely reach your destination. May you find the happiness and fulfillment that you are seeking for there.'"

We asked, "But what if they are going somewhere with bad intentions?"

Gen-la smiled and replied, "That's not your business! This meditation is to develop your own mind. As you generate the mind that
wishes that others will realize their goals and find the satisfaction
they are seeking, you will create the conditions in your own life that
will most assure that your own aspirations will be fulfilled."

Though this driving meditation practice is easy to describe, it is challenging to do! Many times, driving down the road we would begin this practice, only to find that we were many miles or hours down the road before
we realized that we had become distracted. Some days we'd be lost in our
thoughts and forget about doing the meditation at all, and not realize it
until we were hopping on a plane or walking into a meeting.

Just like any meditation practice, when you notice that your attention has
wandered, gently smile to yourself, take a deep breath, and refocus your
mind back into the meditation that you are doing. With meditation practice,
as in other aspects of our lives, sometimes when our practice falls short of
our own expectations or standards it awakens a stronger aspiration and commitment to being more disciplined and mindful. Drive mindfully—radiant
with loving-kindness to your fellow travelers.

28 THE FOUR
IMMEASURABLE ATTITUDES ▼ ▼ ▼

In this classic meditation practice one cultivates the contemplation of immeasurably vast love, compassion, sympathetic joy, and equanimity, and extends these toward all living beings throughout the vastness of time and space.

Consider *love* as the wish that all beings be happy, *compassion* as the wish that all be free from suffering, *sympathetic joy* as an attitude that rejoices in the good fortune of others, and *equanimity* as an attitude of impartiality (not indifference) that regards all beings as essentially equal.

Begin by generating the immeasurably vast attitude of equanimity, recognizing the essential equality and similarity of all beings. Consider how everyone wishes to have happiness and well-being as well as to avoid suffering and pain. Now, in a boundless way, extend the thought: "If all beings were to live in an immeasurable equanimity evenminded and openhearted to all, how wonderful that would be! May all beings come to abide in this evenminded and openhearted state by realizing their essential equality! I will realize this essential equality of all beings and help others to do the same."

Generating an immeasurably vast attitude of love, consider how you yourself and all others wish for happiness. In a boundless way extend the thought: "If all beings were happy and had the causes for happiness, how wonderful that would be! May they come to have this happiness, and may I develop the ability to bring them to happiness."

Generating an immeasurably vast attitude of compassion, consider the many kinds of suffering, pain, and disease experienced by different types of people and other living creatures. In a boundless way extend the wish: "If all beings were free from suffering and the causes of suffering, how wonderful it would be! May they come to be free from their suffering, and may I develop the wisdom and power to be able to free them."

Generating an immeasurably vast attitude of sympathetic joy, consider the positive potentials of all beings. In a boundless way extend the thought: "If all beings were to know the joy of understanding and realizing all their positive potentials, how wonderful that would be. May they come to realize everything that is wonderful! I will help them to realize the causes of true joy!"

Once you have a feeling for the practice, simply allow your mind to settle deeply into the contemplation of each of these qualities. One by one, imagine your love, compassion, rejoicing, and evenminded openheartedness filling the vastness of space extending to all beings everywhere.

As you breathe naturally, bring your awareness to the flow of sensations and the rhythms of your breathing. Notice how each breath—when you attend to it properly—reveals itself as a teacher of change and impermanence, freedom, flow, and the interconnectedness of all beings and all creation.

Notice how with each exhalation, you release and offer a part of yourself to the world, and how with each inhalation you are presented with a gift so precious that it sustains your very life. When the time comes that you breathe out and don't breathe in again, this life will end. Cherish every breath as precious and know each is worthy of your attention. As you breathe, sense that you are breathing with all those beings around you. Contemplate that you are breathing with your loved ones and with your friends…breathing with the strangers passing by…breathing with your coworkers and colleagues…breathing with all the creatures near and far, and with the plants and trees around you that transform the carbon dioxide that you exhale into their own bodies and offer life-giving oxygen in return.

Riding the ever changing waves of your breath, imagine all beings within the atmospheric envelope of our precious planet. With each breath, each being weaves itself into the fabric of life and affirms its kinship with all living beings. Breathing together with all beings, offer each breath as a wave of blessings. Contemplate how, miraculously, the atmosphere of the planet contains approximately the same volume of air as the number of breaths that have ever been breathed. And within each breath are approximately the same number of atoms of oxygen, nitrogen, carbon dioxide, and other molecules as there are the number of breaths in the atmosphere. Thus, in a sense, with each breath, you breathe in billions of molecules of air plus the inspiration of all beings who have ever breathed upon this earth!

Imagine: 22,000 breaths a day, for a lifetime—perhaps 720 billion breaths! In a very real sense, with each breath, you receive into yourself some of the same air that was breathed by every great being who has every walked upon this earth:

▼▼ You breathe with Jesus and Mary.
   You breathe with the Buddha.
   You breathe with Abraham and Sarah, Isaac and Ishmael.
   You breathe with Mohammed...and Joan of Arc...and
   Milarepa...and King Ashoka.
   You breathe with Plato, Newton, and Einstein...
   with Ben Franklin and Black Elk...
   with Confucious and Lao Tsu, Rumi, Saint Francis, and the
   Baal Shem Tov.
   You breathe with the Dalai Lama and the Pope...
   with Gandhi, Martin Luther King, Jr., Nelson Mandela,
   and Mother Theresa...
   with Dorothy Day, Emma Goldman, and Leonard Pelletier...
   You breathe with your great-great grandparents,
   and with infinite ancestors reaching back into the depths of time...
   and you send your breath on to be a source of inspiration
   for your great-great grandchildren and generations to come...
   Sensing the presence of these and countless inspiring beings
   of the past, the present, and the future,
   rest in the flow of this exquisite contemplation.

Allow yourself to become even more attentive now to the flow of your breath—to the natural receiving and radiating pulse of each precious breath. Mindful of yourself breathing with all beings, consider the possibility that with each breath you can draw the inspiration that you most need in this moment, and in this situation—or in any moment and any situation.

Imagine that the intentions you hold in mind, the prayers and yearnings of your heart, and the challenges of the situations you are facing all blend to tune your consciousness and your energy system to resonate with the frequencies and inspirations that are most in tune with your needs in that moment. Whatever you need—peace, clarity, strength, courage, hope—imagine that as you breathe, you can be inspired by those qualities. It's like when you drop a stone in a pool, and the ripples go out to the very edge of that space and then ripple back again to the center where the original impulse began in a way that completes and fulfills the initial impulse.

As you inhale, pause to sense and envision the billions of atoms of air soaking into your bloodstream and being carried to nourish, energize, and truly bless every cell and fiber of you body. As you exhale, pause to envision that through the power of your prayerful intent and imagination you imbue the energy bundles of each atom and molecule of air with the signature frequencies that carry your unique blessings. Imagine the offering of your breath turning the trees greener, sweetening their fruit, and bringing joy to everyone who is touched by your offerings. Envision that each breath is offered as a blessing to the countless beings who will have the good fortune to breathe with you in the moments and ages to come upon this vast and precious world. Let yourself become a great cosmic air purifier, purifying any negative energies held in the air you breathe and offering a bundle of blessings to all beings with each exhalation.

As you rise from this meditation and move on to other activities, allow the ever flowing waves of breath to remind you of this contemplation and invite you to continue to breathe with and for all beings, receiving and radiating with each breath.

▼▼ We appeal to all the inhabitants of this planet. Each cannot be changed for the better unless the consciousness of individuals is changed. We pledge to work for such transformation in individual and collective consciousness, for the awakening of our spiritual powers through reflection, meditation, prayer, or positive thinking, for a conversion of the heart. Together we can move mountains. Without a willingness of taking risks and a readiness to sacrifice there can be no fundamental change in our situation. Therefore, we commit ourselves to a common global ethic, to better mutual understanding, and to socially beneficial, peace-fostering, and Earth-friendly ways of life.

Excerpt from *Toward a Global Ethic*

Wisdom is intuitive knowledge of the mind of love and clarity that lies
beneath one's ego driven anxieties and aggressions. Meditation is
going into the mind to see this for yourself—over and over again, until
it becomes the mind you live in!

Gary Snyder

Of all the meditations for healing that we know of, this meditation
of energy transformation is without equal in its universally practical applications. Its power lies in reaffirming our dynamic interrelationship with all of life, awakening our generative capabilities, and
activating a genuine heartfelt concern for the well-being of others.

When we are physically, emotionally, or mentally suffering, there is a
strong tendency to withdraw from the world and to implode into a very
self-centered and self-protective state. The greater our sense of isolation, the
greater our suffering. This cuts us off from the flow of healing energies that
are available to us. The practice of this meditation helps us to build our
capacity to transform every experience that we may have into an affirmation
of loving concern for ourselves, others, and the world.

As a foundation for this practice, begin by establishing a sense of your
spaciousness using the hollow body meditation (p. 138–41). Then, in the
region of your heart center, imagine a transformational vortex. As you
inhale, imagine drawing into this vortex any mental or physical pain, discomfort or negativity that you may be presently feeling, or any latencies
for future sufferings—envisioning these as dark smoke or as heavy, hot
energy. Imagine that the negative energy is completely dissolved and

transformed within this center.

Now as you exhale, imagine that from your heart center waves of clear, radiant, healing light pour forth. Imagine these waves blazing forth filling your whole body and mind, healing, energizing, and transforming you. Allow this vortex at your heart to function as an energy transformer drawing in negativity, darkness, or pain, and transforming it into radiant light and healing energy. For example, drawing in agitation, radiate peace; drawing in anger, radiate patience and compassion. Allow each breath to deepen and affirm your energetic nature and transformational capabilities.

The healing power of this meditation is really activated when you begin to understand that the radius of your transformational influence can be vast in its scope and that you are able to receive and transform the energies of others in the world around you. The larger the field of interrelationship that you acknowledge and participate in, the greater will be the reservoir of healing energies that you will tap into.

If you are tormented by anger or grief, imagine and affirm that, as you transform these energies or feelings within your own life, the same feelings shared by others are transformed as well. Envision and affirm that a radiance of healing energies radiates out through you to be received by anyone who shares the same feelings. Whatever the form of your distress, use it to affirm the universality of your humanity and your relationship to countless others who might share the same feelings or concerns.

This is a meditation you can do anywhere, under any circumstances. Practice this method quietly and invisibly—as you walk down the street, as you watch the news or witness the chaos in the world—as an active way of transforming negativity and bringing peace and healing into the world.

Keep in mind that your ability to visibly transform the negativities of the world is secondary to transforming the illusion of your own sense of separateness. The real power of this practice lies in developing a deeper experience of kinship with the world, and in breaking free from our preoccupation with our own personal situation. Taken to heart, each breath becomes an affirmation of relatedness and a gesture of compassion.

31 MEDITATION ON THE ANGEL
OF UNIVERSAL COMPASSION ▼ ▼ ▼

The Tibetan word for Buddha is Sang-gye. Sang indicates a state purified of all faults and weaknesses; and gye refers to the expansion of
wisdom to the limits of existence. In that we all have a certain degree
of purity and knowledge, one might say that we are all Buddhas of
varying sizes. Although the Buddha in us is still quite small compared
to a fully enlightened one, full Buddhahood is not something we cannot attain. Imperfection can be systematically eliminated from within
the mind, and every quality of realization can be generated through
correct training.

The Dalai Lama

One time when we were with the Dalai Lama at a gathering of Western scientists and philosophers, he explained that whether they
know it or not, each person is a buddha. People who are fully
awakened to their true divine or universal identity are like big buddhas. And,
to the degree that people lack this awareness or confidence, you might say
that their buddhas are smaller. Yet everyone, every living being, carries with
them at the core of their identity, at the core of their sense of self, a quality
or capacity for fully awakening to their true nature and infinite potentials.

In the Tibetan Buddhist tradition, the angel or archetype of universal
compassion is depicted as having one thousand arms that reach out into the
world to help beings wherever there is suffering. At the end of each of these
arms is a hand, and in the palm of each of these hands is an eye. The hands
reaching out represent the impulse of universal compassion reaching out to

help beings wherever there is pain or suffering or need, which awaken this universal impulse. The eye at the center of each of these hands symbolizes the "eye of wisdom." It is pictured as being fully opened to indicate that the impulse of compassion is guided by wisdom. It is said that wherever there is an act of kindness in the world, the energy and inspiration of this great being of universal compassion is present. The Tibetans would describe this as the inspiring energy or presence of Chenrezig, or Avalokiteswara, and they regard the Dalai Lama as a special embodiment of this Angel of Universal Compassion. Another well-known name for this compassionate being is Quan Yin. Christians would refer to the presence of this compassion as Christ, and followers of the Muslim faith would regard this as the mercy (Rachman) and compassion (Rahim) of Allah.

As a creative or generative meditation, visualize or imagine yourself as an actual embodiment or emanation of this great universal presence—a conduit for this universal loving-kindness to flow into the world as a wave of blessings for all the beings who may be touched by the activities of your body, your speech, and your mind. Imagine how you would live, act, relate, and move through the world if you were to hold yourself as truly an embodiment of this universal being. Generating and activating this enlightened potential within you, allow the presence of suffering within your life—and in the lives of other living beings in the world around you—to open your heart and mind to a quality of compassion that is truly universal in nature.

Taking this contemplation to heart in a disciplined way is a meditation practice that is at the heart and core of many of the world's great mystical traditions. The fruits of such a meditative discipline awaken within us a sense of what is sometimes described as "divine pride," or "sacred dignity," which is a state of the utmost humility and reverence, yet one of faith in the sacred presence of our truest deepest nature.

▼▼ There is a light in this world, a healing spirit more powerful than any darkness we may encounter. We sometimes lose sight of this force when there is suffering, too much pain. Then suddenly, the spirit will emerge through the lives of ordinary people who hear a call and answer in extraordinary ways.

Mother Theresa

Do not believe in what you have heard; do not believe in the traditions because they have been handed down for generations; do not believe in anything because it is rumored or spoken by many, do not believe merely because a written statement of some old sage is produced; do not believe in conjectures; do not believe in that as truth to which you have become attached by habit; do not believe merely the authority of your teachers and elders. After observation and analysis, when it agrees with reason and is conducive to the good and gain of one and all, then accept it, practice it and live up to it.

The Buddha

This meditation is drawn from *Silent Mind, Holy Mind* by Lama Thubten Yeshe. As a daily practice, you could do the following. Sit, or kneel if you like, in a comfortable position, relaxed but with your back straight. In your mind's eye, visualize Jesus (or any other great teacher or spiritual friend) before you. His face has a tranquil, peaceful, and loving expression. A picture of the resurrected Christ or of Jesus teaching may be used as a model for this visualization.

Then visualize, from the crown of his head, radiant, white light coming to your own crown. This white light is in the nature of blissful energy, and as it enters your body, it purifies the physical contamination, or sin, accumulated over countless lifetimes. This blissful, white energy purifies all diseases of the body and activates and renews the functioning of your entire nervous system.

In a similar manner, red light is visualized radiating forth from Jesus' throat and entering your own, completely pervading your vocal center with the sensation of bliss. If you have difficulties with your speech—always telling lies, being uncontrolled in what you say, engaging in slander, using harsh language or the like—this blissful red energy purifies you of all these negativities. As a result you discover the divine qualities of speech.

Then from Jesus' heart, infinite radiant blue light comes to sink into your heart, purifying your mind of all its wrong conceptions. Your selfish and petty ego, which is like the chief or president of the delusions, and the three poisons of greed, hatred, and ignorance, which are like the ego's ministers, are all purified in this blissful blue radiance. The indecisive mind, which is especially doubtful and caught between "maybe this" and "maybe that," is clarified. Also purified is the narrow mind, which cannot see the totality, because its focus is too tight. As the light energy fills your mind, your heart becomes like the blue sky, embracing universal reality and all of space.

This three-part purification of body, speech, and mind can be very helpful for anyone with great devotion to Jesus. If you are unable to visualize all of the above, you can concentrate merely on Jesus' heart. From this center very blissful white, radiant energy comes to your heart, purifying all defilements. This is a simplified practice, but still can be extremely helpful.

You can conclude this meditation by visualizing a white lotus flower blooming in your heart. The compassionate figure visualized in front of you then sinks into your heart and manifests on this lotus seat. Afterward, whatever you eat or drink becomes an offering to this Jesus within your heart. If this meditation is done daily with good concentration and a pure motivation, it can be very effective in transforming your ordinary actions, words, and thoughts and in bringing you closer to the divine qualities of Jesus.

▼▼ Silent meditation, without thought, totally open,
awake and aware, this is absolute prayer!
Lama Thubten Yeshe

The following meditation was told to John Blofeld by an old woman, a
nun, in Canton.

You sit down on a hilltop, or anywhere high enough
for you to see nothing but the sky in front of your eyes.
With your mind you make everything empty.

There is nothing there you say.
And you see it like that—nothing
emptiness.

Then you say *ahhh*...
But there *is* something!
Look there's the sea
and the moon has risen
full, round, white.

And you see it like that
sea, silver in the moonlight
with little white topped waves.
And in the blue black sky above
hangs a great moon
bright,
but not dazzling,
a soft brightness you might say.

You stare at the moon a long
long time, feeling calm, happy.
Then the moon gets smaller,
but brighter and brighter and brighter
till you see it as a pearl, or a seed, but so bright
you can only just bear to look at it.

The pearl starts to grow.
And before you know what's happened,
it's Kuan Yin, the Mother of Compassion, herself
standing up against the sky
all dressed in gleaming white
and with her feet resting on a lotus
that floats on the waves.

You see her
once you know how to do it
as clearly as I see you.
Her robes are shining,
and there's a halo round her head.
She smiles at you,
such a loving smile. She's so glad
to see you that tears of happiness sparkle in her eyes.
If you keep your mind calm,
by just whispering her name
and not trying too hard she will stay a long time.

When she does go,
it's by getting smaller and smaller.
She doesn't go back to being a pearl,
but just gets so small
that at last you can't see her, then you notice
that the sky and sea
have vanished too.

Just space is left.
Lovely, lovely space, going on forever...

that space stays long
if you can do without *you*. Not *you* and space, you see

just space.

No you!

Sitting quietly with your eyes closed or slightly open, imagine a luminous sphere of light, like the sun, shining in the space in front and above you. Let this sphere be an idealized representation of all the mental, physical, emotional, and spiritual qualities that you most wish to energize and embody in your life at this time. Vividly imagine that you are soaking up all the rays of this light source and its energy of relaxation, calm, clarity, and inner strength, as though you were sunbathing. Feel these rays soaking into you, pervading your body and mind—more deeply and completely with each breath. Let these feelings of calmness, inner strength, and harmony grow and glow deeply within you.

Now imagine that this shining luminous sphere sends light tendrils out to all corners of the universe, to all the sources of inspiration, healing, and harmonizing energy that you need at this time. Imagine these rays of light drawing back into this sphere all the healing and harmonizing power that exists throughout space and time. It all pours back into your shining sphere of light, charging it up into a crystal that showers you with the light of a billion shining suns. Now imagine this brilliant light energy streaming into you, completely dissolving all your tensions and pains, all your worries and cares, healing and opening the places in your body, heart, and mind that need to become whole. Feel the inner clouds of darkness vanishing in this flood of brilliant light. Feel the fog of sluggishness and dullness dissolve completely into a vitalized calm within.

Imagine this shining sphere of light coming closer now, pouring its light down into you. Let it come to the top of your head. Feel a shower of cleansing, healing, purifying light flooding you, washing you completely clean and clear throughout. Vividly imagine your body as a crystal flooded with rainbow light. Now imagine this light pouring through you, shining through your eyes, from your heart, through the pores of your skin. Flowing out into the world. Tidal waves of healing, helpful, crystal, rainbow-like light shining to you. Flowing through you and into the world.

Now, if you like, imagine this luminous sphere coming down into you like a glorious brilliant nova of powerful rainbow light slipping into a crystal sea, merging and melting into the luminous open space within you. Imagine that it transforms your body and mind into a vast open state of unimpeded clarity and luminosity, and that your emotions are transformed into those of power, harmony, generosity, and confidence.

Experience yourself as a radiant being. Feel this deep vital energy pouring deeply through you and out into the world. Experience the peaceful power of this way of seeing yourself. Imagine that these waves of positive feeling are like clear rainbow light that can reach out to others in ways that bring relief, inspiration, energy, or whatever else they may need. Wherever you direct your attention, let there be benefit.

35 MEDITATIONS FOR DYING ▼ ▼ ▼

We never know which will come first:
Our next breath or
Our next life.

Tibetan proverb

In some contemplative traditions, the practice of meditation is viewed as the supreme vehicle for developing a presence of mind subtle enough so that at the time of your death you can die consciously and thus "navigate" and make choices as to the trajectory of your consciousness. It is taught that the primary training ground for being mindfully present at the time of death is to learn to be mindfully present, or lucid, in your dreams. The training ground for being mindful of your dreams is to develop greater mindfulness in the "waking dream" of your ordinary life.

Though the practice of mindfulness is simple to describe, it is very profound. As you become more present to what is going on within and around you, you will discover doorways to greater freedom in every realm of your being.

In the Tibetan contemplative tradition, meditative practices for transferring consciousness at the time of death are widely practiced. These meditations, called *phowa*, are traditionally practiced by a person at the time of his or her own death, or by others who help the dying direct their consciousness onto a beneficial trajectory at the end of this life. Phowa meditation is often complemented by reflective and generative meditations that simulate the actual dying process.

Over the years, we have learned many versions of these practices from Sogyal Rinpoche, Chagdud Rinpoche, and other precious teachers from this Tibetan tradition. The meditations that follow here are offered as healing meditations for the living and the dying, as well as for those who have already died.

The first step is to calm and quiet your mind, being mindful of your breath or using any of the calming meditations introduced earlier in this book. Then invoke before you the radiant presence of any spiritual figure toward whom you feel a heartfelt sense of devotion and faith. From your heart, pray to this loving, compassionate presence for the blessings, spiritual strength, purification, protection, and inspiration necessary to die a good death and to realize liberation or enlightenment in the dying process.

Next, imagine that this presence of light is so moved by your heartfelt prayer that he or she smiles lovingly and radiates love and compassion as streams of light from his or her heart. As these absorb into you, allow yourself to feel purified of any negative karma, destructive emotional energy, obscurations of mind, or blockages in the subtle energy system that may lead to suffering in the future. See and feel yourself immersed in pure loving light.

Then, allow yourself to dissolve completely into light. Next, imagine your consciousness as a sphere of light at your heart that flashes out from you like a shooting star and flies up into the heart of the radiant spiritual presence in front of you, merging inseparably with this blissful presence of light. Remain in that state of unification with this presence for as long as possible.

Our teachers say that to have the presence of mind to actually use this practice well at the time of death, timing is critical. To accomplish this successfully, they generally recommend performing the phowa practice during the actual onset of the dying process, when the breathing becomes shallower, the pulse weakens, the senses begin to withdraw, and the life-force wanes. Especially during the time of a person's last breaths, this practice can be repeated many times. It is at the time of one's death that one has the opportunity to apply the subtle quality and presence of mind that has been cultivated, ideally, through a lifetime of meditation practice. Yet, even under the best of circumstances at the time of our own dying, it may be very helpful to have a loved one or friend actually guide us through this meditation or other instructions on dying. (See Sogyal Rinpoche's excellent book *The Tibetan Book of Living and Dying* for more guidance.) This practice is traditionally read or whispered gently into the ear of a dying person.

This same meditation can be used to assist others at the time of their death. To accomplish this, remember that the principle is the same, the only difference being that you visualize the spiritual presence above the head of the dying persons, imagine them being purified, dissolving into light and merging into this spiritual presence. If possible, do this practice especially as they are breathing their last breath, or as soon as the breathing stops and before the body is touched or moved. This tradition teaches that there are subtle stages of dying that continue after the breathing has stopped and the heart has stopped beating. It is therefore recommended, if possible, not to move the body, but to keep it still and to continue with the phowa meditation, prayers, and sacred chants for some time after the person has died. If you are unable to be physically with a person, the practice can still be effective from a distance, or even after a person has died. We have heard the lamas teach that it can be effective to do this practice at the place a person has died, and every seventh day after a person has died for seven weeks.

In his inspiring book *The Tibetan Book of Living and Dying* Sogyal Rinpoche describes one way to do this practice: "Simply merge your mind with the wisdom mind of pure presence. Consider: 'My mind and the mind of the Buddha are one.'" He reminds us that "sometimes the most powerful practices can be the most simple," and invites us to practice in this way until it becomes second nature—as the time of our death is uncertain, and we never know when we might need to call upon what we have learned.

Variations on this meditation practice can also be done when you hear on the news that there has been a disaster, as you contemplate the needless deaths of tens of thousands of children each day due to preventable disease and starvation, or even when you stop to consider the millions of lives that are lost each day in the process of slaughtering animals as food for human beings. In such moments, the following visualization meditation can be very helpful:

> From the heart of the Great Being in the sky before you waves
> of rainbow light shine forth throughout all the world and
> through all dimensions, enveloping the beings who have died

wherever they are, purifying their karma, and infusing them with radiant blessings. Their ordinary forms dissolve and they become brilliant spheres of light that are drawn back to dissolve into this Great Being's heart-mind—a realm beyond the cycles of suffering, a realm of absolute purity and bliss.

When you are doing this meditation for people who have died, it is traditionally recommended to meditate in this way during the forty-nine days after their death, and to dedicate the merit of your practice to their ongoing spiritual development and well being.

Finally, if all the details of this meditation elude you at the time of a death, then simply, prayerfully, recite a prayer or mantra that carries a sacred vibration with it during and following the time of passing. If you are Jewish, you might recite the Sh'ma; if you are Christian, the Lord's Prayer; if you are Muslim, the Zikr; if you are a Tibetan Buddhist, the mantra *om mani padme hung* may guide your loving thoughts and add comfort during the passage of death.

Through the parallelism of body, mind and speech, the coordination
of movement, thought and word, the harmony of feeling, creative
imagination, visualization and verbal expression, we achieve a unity
of all the functions of our conscious being, which not only affects the
surface of our personality—namely our senses and our intellect—but
equally the deeper regions of our mind. In the regular performance of
such ritual worship, the very foundations of our being are slowly but
certainly transformed and made receptive for the inner light.

Lama Govinda

One day, as a young boy, when I was in the synagogue with my
grandfather, a very old and pious man came over to say hello. He
had always caught my eye as being a uniquely calm and wise-
looking fellow, and as he approached he seemed to be mumbling serenely
to himself. Coming to stand in front of us, his moving lips softly chanted the
words, "The Lord is good", *Baruch Ha Shem* in Hebrew. He had a short chat
with Gramps, all the while inaudibly chanting this mantra-like phrase over
and over behind and between his words. His final audible words to us were
the same as his first, and as he left he seemed to glide on this mantric wave
as a continuum of steadiness and balance for his mind.

Over the years, we've been introduced to the use of mantra or chanting
in every meditative tradition that we've studied. The actual Sanskrit word
mantra means "mind protection." That is to say that while one is engaged in
chanting a mantra, one's mind is protected from dissipating its clarity and
power in random or negative thoughts. In many meditative traditions,

formal periods of quiet contemplative practice are preceded by a time of devotional chanting or mantric repetition. The repetitive and often sacred nature of these chants can have a calming and stabilizing effect that builds coherence and power in the mind and the subtle nervous system.

The use of such mind protectors is an old sacred science. The inner scientist knows and understands the use of sound and vibration as a tool to evoke and refine specific qualities of mind. In Native American traditions a young man or woman would be sent on a vision quest and told to listen for a sacred song or death chant that the Great Spirit would teach them during this time of alert, receptive vigilance. After days of fasting, prayer, or other ordeals, a chant would emerge into awareness as a gift or sign from the Great Spirit. From that time on, this death chant would be used to steady and protect the mind at critical times in one's life. Having practiced this chant in the face of adversity possibly millions of times over the course of one's life, one would turn to it wholeheartedly and single-pointedly as one approached the moment of death, allowing it to carry one across the threshold between worlds and into the vastness of Spirit.

In the Tibetan tradition, the repetition of the mantras *om mani padme hung, om ah hung vajra guru padma siddhi hung,* and *om tare tuttare ture svaha* are commonly recited 100,000 to 100 million times in the course of one's life. The subtle psychophysical repetition of such mantric practice provides one with a coherent internal resonance that pervades one's mindbody as well as a continual sense of direct connection with the source of spiritual blessings, power, and inspiration. The power of mantras, some say, is related to the use. cumulative effect of countless conscious repetitions over millennia of their By chanting a mantra, one's mindbody sympathetically resonates with the cosmic reservoir of its accumulated power, and if properly receptive, one will experience an infusion of the blessing energy of that particular mantra.

Clinically we've introduced this meditative practice to people who need to quiet and gentle their minds, with pregnant women and dying patients and loved ones. A friend who is an anesthesiologist often chants mantras in his patients ears as they drift off on the anesthetic. Throughout a pregnancy, a woman or couple can chant a mantra or sing a song of particular beauty or feeling for them. Gradually the fetus will become imbued with this familiar resonance. After birth, this can be chanted to them as a lullaby of reassurance, reducing the trauma of the birth transition. It can also be taught to other members of the family and babysitters as a sound of comfort from across the room. Children will often respond in an alert and responsive way to these familiar sounds from their time in the womb.

The mantra *om mani padme hung* has been a final lullaby easing the transition of death for many special loved ones and friends. In the last days of their life, when there wasn't much to say in words, the gentle audible presence of this or other mantras effectively brought balance to their minds as they moved to subtler and subtler states of consciousness.

One of our wisest and kindest teachers, a true master of meditation who has spent nearly a third of his eighty-two years in various contemplative retreats, is continually chanting mantras as he directs his attention and intention of blessing toward countless beings. Used in this way, repetition of mantra is mental target practice in which all living beings are the targets of a heartfelt intention that is projected and carried by the mantra. Christian practitioners might chant the name of Jesus or say hallelujah, Hebrew practitioners chant the *Sh'ma* or say shalom, Sufis the Zikar; others might work with *om*, love, peace, joy, or other such things. Though there is power in the actual vibration and sound of traditional mantras, the mental intention in its use determines the power and magnitude of its benefit.

The actual practice of mantra meditation can be quite simple. You can just sit quietly and mentally recite a mantra or meaningful phrase, resting the mind upon its sound or its inner resonance within you. Whenever your mind wanders, simply return to the repetition and keep your attention on what you are doing. To elaborate on this method, visualize waves of light and healing vibrations pouring from your heart to others, bringing more light, love, and happiness into the world, and dissolving the darkness, pain, and fear that fills the minds of so many beings.

When you have a feeling for it, working with a mantra can help to calm and focus the mind when you are busy in the world. It is a simple, effective method for strengthening and developing positive qualities of the mind in moments that are ordinarily wasted—driving to work, waiting in line, holding the line on a telephone, walking down the street, and so on: all ordinary activities that can be easily integrated into your meditation practice.

The practice of the inner essence of mind protection is more a state of mind than a vocalization. In its deepest essence, it is a state of being that recognizes and affirms the nonduality and interdependent relationship of all beings and things. Realizing this, the aspiration to contribute to the well-being of others spontaneously arises. This aspiration is made manifest not only through kind words and helpful actions, but through a resonance of heart and mind that reaches out to others in a deep, quiet, and loving way.

When the mind is busy or directed toward superficial appearances, simply chanting a mantra with the intention of creating a more positive atmosphere in the world within and around you can be very helpful. As your mind becomes more subtle and quiet, the repetition of the mantra may likewise become subtler and subtler, until you rest in its innermost essence—silent prayer, a way of simply being natural that brings peace to the world within and around you. In this way, mantra and spoken prayer merge into silence and become the prayer of the heart.

▼▼ This garden universe vibrates complete
Some may hear a sound so sweet.
Vibration reaching up to become light
And then through gamma, out of sight.
Between the eyes and ears there lie
The sounds of color and the light of a sigh
And to hear the sun, what a thing to believe
But it's all around if we could but perceive.
To know ultraviolet, infrared and x-rays
Beauty to find in so many ways.
Two notes of the chord, that's our forescope
And to reach that chord is our life's hope
And to name the chord is important to some
So they give it a word
And that word is
om
Moody Blues

From every human being there arises a light that reaches straight to heaven. And when two souls destined to be together find each other, their streams of light flow together and a single, brighter light goes forth from their united being.

Baal Shem Tov

Sharing meditation time can be a powerful means of bringing depth and aliveness to our relationships. Meditating with a partner provides an opportunity to let our conceptual and emotional dust clear in order to see each other clearly, freshly, and in the ever unfolding newness of each moment. Though an entire volume could be devoted to the intricacies and delicacies of these dyadic meditations, we will briefly describe some ideas or techniques that you might enjoy exploring with a special friend.

1. ATTUNEMENT

Sit across from your partner palm to palm with your left hands facing upward and your right hands facing downward. Take a few moments to breathe, relax, clear, and open your minds. As you breathe begin to establish and energize a sense of your center of energy, awareness, and heartfulness. Using your breathing, begin to extend a field or sphere of these feelings and vibrations around you as you envelop your partner. Simultaneously sense and allow the field and presence of your partner to be ever more deeply within and around you. Allow your fields of luminously charged awareness to blend into a field of sympathetic and harmonious resonance as though the two notes of your spirits were reaching out to merge into a chord of shared awareness.

2. BREATH SYNCHRONY

A. While your partner sits quietly in meditation, bring your attention to the rhythm of your partner's breathing. Gradually allow yourself to come into sync with their breathing. Coming into resonance, empathize.

B. This time simultaneously bring your attention to each other's breathing. Gradually allow your rhythms of inhaling and exhaling to come together. Let this shared attunement bring you into greater harmony and understanding at deeper and deeper levels.

3. GIVING AND RECEIVING

Alternate inhalations and exhalations with your partner. Imagine breathing out love, energy, light, or healing energy to your partner as your partner breathes that in. As you breathe in allow yourself to receive whatever quality of heart or mind they send to you. Let this method teach you about how you can open your heart and mind to both give and receive more generously.

4. MERGING HEARTS AND MIND

With your partner, contemplate and feel the denseness and solidity of your bodies. Next shift your attention to a subtler body of energy, vibration, and movement within this dense and solid form. At an even subtler level, sense an inner openness, spaciousness, and boundlessness, like a vast inner sky that pervades your whole form and energy patterning. In the dimension of form we merge sexually. In the dimension of energy and vibration we communicate and sense resonance, dissonance, and emotions. In the dimension of our openness we are of one essence interpenetrating and pervading all and sharing an open space of mind.

Within this matrix of form-energy-space, establish a nucleus or center of love and luminously positive feelings. From this center you might physically reach out to your partner with a physical caress, a kind word. At the level of vibration, your communication may be as a luminous wave of love and caring. Imagine and sense the possibility of your spheres of energy and space merging and interpenetrating. Though your bodies occupy distinct spaces, imagine what it would feel like if your spheres of energy and openness could interpenetrate. Allow your centers to merge and your fields of energy and awareness to become completely shared. Intimately feel within each other. From your heart, fill your partner with love, and offer energy to your partner to use as he or she most needs it at this time. From your hearts share the flow of unspoken yet profoundly intimate communication springing from the depths of your hearts and minds. After a while gradually breathe your awareness back into its ordinary form-energy-space matrix and rejoice in the deep intimate sense of unity and wholeness that you have shared.

This is an excellent meditation to use to extend healing or love to a loved one who may be far away. When we are apart from each other we choose a time to meditate together in this way each day, and at other times we will drop in for a visit or just to say, "I love you." With practice you will learn to intimately sense and integrate these three dimensions of aliveness within you. As you bring more attention to the dynamic interplay of form-energy-openness in your life, this inner wisdom will become more apparent and will enrich the quality of your relationships as well.

The following meditation can open the way to a direct and profound insight into the nature of mind and perceived phenomena. Envision a luminous sphere spontaneously and effortlessly appearing in the space before you. Allow its luminous clarity to pervade the surrounding space with a sense of both luminous clarity and "knowingness."

Next, envision similar spheres of luminous knowingness spontaneously and naturally emerging from the space above and below and to either side of the original sphere, thus forming a cluster of five. Now envision that each of these secondary spheres becomes the center of another cluster of five. Then allow each of these spheres to become a nucleus of further multiples of this fivefold patterning. Continue to multiply these lights out in clusters of four spheres, each of which becomes a nucleus for a further cluster, until the whole space is pervaded by a unified field of luminous knowingness.

Another approach to this meditation is to envision a sphere of luminous knowingness spontaneously arising at your own center of mindbody. Sense and feel its luminous knowingness pervading the whole space within and around you. Envision in the field of space surrounding you that similar spheres of luminous clarity emerge before you, behind you, to your left and right, as well as above and below you. Each of these spheres is identical and all together they form a matrix of seven with six clustered around the central sphere. Beginning with the sphere before you, envision this sphere now becoming the center of a similar cluster with six around it. Then one by one allow each of the primary spheres around you to become the center of a new cluster, a higher order of luminous knowing spheres. Continue to multiply these lights out in clusters of six spheres, each of which become the nucleus for a further cluster, until the whole space within and surrounding you is pervaded by a unified matrix of knowing luminosity. Bring an effortless and quietly joyful mind to this meditation. Avoid struggling or trying too hard to get it right, but simply practice again and again until it becomes effortless to multiply these luminous spheres and establish this matrix of mind.

Practice dissolving yourself and the world into this unified clarity. As sights, sounds, colors, and other phenomena begin to emerge within and around you, allow each new experience whether sensory or mental to be regarded as a spontaneous, selfless, creative play of mind.

Through this meditation you may come to know mind as intimately pervading and unifying the field of your experience. Within this matrix of mind, know that you can loosen your need for an "I" or experiencer that stands separate from others and from perceived objects. Though appearances may continue to appear distinct and separate from you, gradually the practice of this meditation will reveal that the nature of mind, and the world it perceives, is actually nondual and intimately related.

▼▼ The tower is as wide and spacious as the sky itself. The ground is paved with (innumerable) precious stones of all kinds and there are within the tower (innumerable) palaces, porches, windows, staircases, railings and passages all of which are made of the seven kinds of precious gems.

And within this tower, spacious and exquisitely ornamented, there are hundreds of thousands…of towers each one of which is as exquisitely ornamented as the main tower itself and as spacious as the sky.

And all of the towers, beyond calculation in number, stand not at all in one another way, each preserves its individual existence in perfect harmony with all the rest…there is a state of perfect intermingling and yet of perfect orderliness. Sudhanan, the young pilgrim, sees himself in all the towers as well as in each single tower where all is contained in one and each contains all.

Avatamsaka Sutra

How do we know if our practice is a real practice?
Only by one thing: more and more, we just see the wonder.
What is the wonder? I don't know.
We can't know such things through thinking.
But we always know it when it's there.

Charlotte Joko Beck

Waking up: As you awaken in the morning, in your first conscious moment, wiggle your toes or look at your hands. With wonder and gratitude, awaken to acknowledge the many gifts of this new day—hands that are able to perform the most intricate movements, toes that wiggle, and eyes, ears, and other faculties that enable you to behold this most amazing world. If you awaken with a loved one, give them a cuddle and appreciate the gift he or she is to you.

Aspiration: Then contemplate and ask yourself, "How do I want to live this day?" Generate a heartfelt and sincere aspiration that affirms the quality of presence and action that you yearn to bring alive today. Then, throughout the day check and renew your intention.

Reflection and dedication: In the evening before you are too tired, or before bed, reflect upon how you have lived and what you have learned today. Consider how often and how well you remembered and stayed true to the aspiration you generated in the morning, and reflect upon what you have learned through your successes and stumbles throughout the day.

Imagine gathering all the positive energies and learnings that you experienced throughout the day and dedicating the benefit of your practice to your continued spiritual development and to the well-being and awakening of all. Then, before going to sleep, generate a heartfelt aspiration/prayer for the morrow, and follow with one of the sleeping meditations. (See pp. 120–21.)

FIVE STEPS FOR A DAILY MEDITATION PRACTICE

The following simple guidelines can help you to establish a daily meditation practice that allows room for some variety and richness. With practice, this simple flow of methods will become quite natural, and your confidence in weaving these pieces together will grow. There are five parts to this sequence:

1. *Inspiration and Intention:* As you begin, take a short time to clarify your intention and offer a prayer of gratitude or a call for inspiration. Remembering that meditation is the practice of deep relationship, and that you never practice "alone," call upon the sources of inspiration in your life, that they may guide and inspire your meditation. Remembering all those who share your life and world, practice in order to in some way become a force of healing and wholeness in the world.
2. *Concentration:* Next, shift to practice some type of focusing, concentration meditation such as mindfulness of breathing, or the nine-part breath, or the elemental breaths.
3. *Meditation:* Then shift to a longer period of quiet meditation using whatever technique you are drawn to.
4. *Dedication:* Finally, end the session with a brief dedication, gathering the potency generated through this time of meditation into your heart and radiating it to share the blessings with all beings.
5. *Application:* As you conclude your formal meditation practice, make a smooth transition and hold the intention to carry this quality of mindful presence into whatever activities will follow. Throughout the day, pause from time to time for a mini-meditation to renew your connection to these qualities, and then continue to infuse your life with the mindful presence, insight, creativity, and compassion that flow from your formal meditation time.

Though these five phases build upon each other, if time or inclination do not permit, you will still find benefit in doing only 1, 2 and 4, or 1 and 2, or even just 1! Give yourself credit for any sincere steps that you make in the right direction.

Keep your formal practice short and simple at first so that you can begin to establish this new life pattern and feel some success in maintaining it. Then, as you see the benefits, gradually develop, deepen, or expand your meditation practice.

WEAVING MEDITATION INTO OUR LIVES AND WORK

There are many simple ways to weave these practices of meditation into your daily life. For example, one woman we know does the nine-part breath every morning while waiting for her car to warm up. Another friend makes it a daily ritual to watch the sun come up and to contemplate his life in relationship to the cosmos. Others take time each day for contemplative prayer. Many friends practice mindful walking on the way to work. For others, reading or listening to the morning news and opening their hearts to send healing prayers to those suffering throughout the world is a daily form of meditation. Some people practice mindfulness of breathing to polish their minds, or mindfully watch the creative display of the mind's amazing potential.

Some people find it helpful to practice loving-kindness meditation on the way to and from work, radiating wishes of peace, happiness, health, and protection to all the drivers rushing headlong around them. Others recite mantras or prayers to steady and anchor themselves in a deeper rhythm as they drive or walk to work. For some of us, a morning meditation may simply be the practice of "mindful shaving," mindful makeup application, or mindful eating of breakfast before launching off into a busy day. If you exercise in the mornings, we encourage you to build in an extra five to twenty minutes at the end of your workout to practice deep relaxation and meditation. As mentioned earlier, the physiological rebound into deep relaxation after exercise can also be an especially good time to deeply relax and meditate—at whatever time of the day that might be.

One final strategy is to let your conversations and interactions with people throughout the day become opportunities to practice deep listening and mindful speaking. Even if you only transform a few encounters throughout the day with a meditative quality of presence, this will still be quite revolutionary. Approached in this way, with awareness and compassion, every activity of your daily life can become a vehicle to deepen your meditation.

GETTING STARTED

Because mindlessness and distraction are such well-established habits, any movement toward developing a meditation practice is a step in the right direction. Most people don't feel they have the time to add meditation to the long list of "duties" already crowding their daily life. As a starting point, we suggest that you experiment with simply being mindful as you do something you regularly do every day, or something that you enjoy. For instance, if you like to walk, walk mindfully. If you like to listen to music, then give yourself time to really listen to some music. If you like to take showers or bubble baths, then bathe mindfully. Or, as you talk with someone whom you love, read a story to your child, or make love with your lover, really be there wholeheartedly in the experience.

You can also transform other everyday experiences into meditations. Experiment with mindfully centering yourself by inhaling and exhaling three times at each red stop light, for example. Simple things—brushing your teeth, walking to your office, or mindfully tasting and chewing the first three mouthfuls of food at each meal—can all become opportunities to practice being present. Following those few mindful moments, carry that quality of attention into whatever activity comes next. See how many of the mindless moments of your day can be transformed into opportunities to strengthen concentration, develop mindfulness, deepen insight, expand creativity, and open your heart. Every activity and every moment of the day offers an invitation to open the door of your heart-mind to a deeper quality of aliveness, relationship, and inspiration.

Though quality attention is important for the actual time of your meditation, remember that the real goal of meditation practice is to develop a quality of lucid, loving, peaceful, radiant presence that you can then carry over into every moment of your life. Formal meditation time is really just an opportunity to practice, without distraction, bringing alive the qualities and ways of being you hope to awaken more fully in the other moments of your day.

PART FOUR
▼ ▼ ▼ CONTEMPLATIVE WISDOM
IN DAILY LIFE

Everything we do—our discipline, effort, meditation,
livelihood, and every single thing we do from the moment
we're born until the moment we die—we can use to help us
to realize our unity and our completeness with all things.

Pema Chödron

1 DEEPENING YOUR MEDITATION PRACTICE ▼ ▼ ▼

CULTIVATING MOMENTUM

Though there is some advantage in practicing meditation now and then, the real benefits come through establishing the discipline and momentum of daily practice. This is analogous to physical training. Intermittent exercise may feel good on occasion, but does little to condition the body or to develop strength, health, or vitality. Similarly, sporadic meditation practice may feel good but offers little benefit compared to daily practice. An ongoing meditation practice increases the power of your presence and the focus of your attention, and it strengthens your mindbody. Over time the sustained practice of meditation enhances myriad capacities for bringing a deeper clarity, responsiveness, resilience, wisdom, and creativity to life. During our many years of laboratory research on meditation we have seen measurable changes in brain function in experienced meditators, and this has deeply inspired us to practice these methods. Over the past thirty plus years we have witnessed the development and maturation of thousands of meditators who have stayed with the practice. Having known them in the past, and seeing who they have become, we are often impressed by how profoundly these practices have transformed the quality of these people's lives.

As in the creative arts, spiritual traditions for thousands of years have recognized the value of disciplined practice. Although people might have a talent or latent potential, without discipline they can't cultivate it. Developing the discipline and momentum of an ongoing meditation practice can help you to generate the inner strength, resilience, self-confidence, insight, and faith necessary to support you during difficult times. Without such discipline, every time you begin again is like starting from scratch, with little foundation, depth, or momentum to draw upon.

THE WISDOM OF SABBATH

Daily meditation or worship, observance of the Sabbath, times of pilgrimage, vision quest, or contemplative retreat have been integral ways of life for people and cultures to stay tapped into the wellsprings of inspiration that continually revitalize their lives. All contemplative traditions encourage their followers to make time in their busy lives to deepen their meditation practice and to contemplate the teachings. Traditionally, every year has periods devoted to retreat and meditation, every week has a Sabbath or day of mindfulness, and every day has special times for specific meditations or prayers.

For the Jewish people, the Sabbath is a time when the spirit of the Shechina—a feminine aspect of the Divine—most fully dwells within and among us. For twenty-four glorious hours we simplify our lives in order to abide in communion, sanctified and blessed with this mysterious presence, remembering, affirming, and celebrating the deep, subtle, and universal dimensions and mysteries of our being that we so easily forget during our busy weekday lives. As the Sabbath ends, we dedicate ourselves to keeping this spirit alive as we launch back into the complexity of our lives and work in the world.

Throughout our busy lives and work, in every moment that we pause to collect ourselves, to relax our bodies, to focus our minds, or to meditate, we create a Sabbath moment. In these moments of meditation practice we invite the mindlessness, insensitivity, turbulence, distraction, and dullness of our daily lives to depart, and we invite the spirit of peaceful, lucid, loving, radiant presence to come forth and abide within us. Such moments are in a sense sanctified and blessed by the presence that we cultivate and carry with us. It is in these moments that we are able return to a state of being that affirms our true nature and potentials, and that draws inspiration from center, source, Sabbath, wilderness, mystery, and spirit that is reflected within us.

GUIDELINES FOR DAYS OF CONTEMPLATIVE RETREAT

It is very helpful to occasionally dedicate a longer period of time to developing and deepening your meditation practice. Setting aside a morning or a day or even a weekend or a week for a meditation retreat can provide an inspiring oasis amid the compression and intensity of your busy life. Since the time will be hard to "find," we suggest that you *make* the time, knowing that you will return from this "time on the mountain"—even if you've never left your own home—with renewed inspiration and insight to guide your busy daily life.

Here are some guidelines for creating a day of mindfulness and meditation. Let this be a day of Sabbath—of deep reflection, rest, and spiritual renewal, a day when you turn off the phone, stay out of your email, and simplify your life so that you focus on what really has heart, soul, and meaning for you. Let this be a day when you can devote your complete undivided attention to developing and deepening your meditation practice.

Just as you might choose a piece or two of music in order to learn how to play really well, or have a software program that may take you some time to master, as you prepare for this day, select one, two, or three meditations that you would like to deepen your connection with. If you like, you can also select some inspirational readings from other sources and set up some pictures of loved ones or teachers who inspire you. It's helpful to create an inspiring physical environment by cleaning and clearing the space for your retreat and setting up flowers, candles, or perhaps some music that might be uplifting between your meditation sessions.

As you begin your retreat, clarify your intention for this special time. Remind yourself why this is an important time for you, and what it is that you want to focus on. Dedicate yourself to deepening the wisdom and love you bring to life, and to the lives of all whose lives you touch.

Also set an intention to approach everything that you do today—your sitting meditation, walking, bathing, even going to the toilet or preparing and eating food—as a mindful meditation. Let the continuity of your mindful awareness weave every moment of this day into your meditation practice.

As you practice, remember to keep your meditation sessions short enough that you can stay focused, and to concentrate on the quality of your meditation not only its sheer duration. Discipline yourself to stay focused on what you are doing and to not let your mind drift into distracting thoughts or to sink into dullness. When you do become distracted, simply refocus on the practice and begin again.

It may be helpful to precede or follow your meditation sessions with some time of walking or stretching meditation, self-massage, or inspirational reading.

If you find that your meditations are being clouded by sleepiness, this may be a sign that you are really exhausted. If this is the case, then it might be most skillful and kind to give yourself permission to take a nap or to go for a long, mindful walking meditation.

If you find that your meditations are being clouded by the recurring intrusion of distracting thoughts about an issue or challenge in your life, then it may be wise to consider focusing on that issue as a "reflective meditation" for a while. (See *Reflective meditation* on p. 131.)

If you like, consider devoting part of your day to a mindful service project that would delight or bring benefit to others. This might be to make or fix something for a loved one or friend, plant some flowers or trees, prepare a meal for someone who is housebound, or help clean up a neighborhood park. Engage in this activity as a mindfulness meditation practice and stay very present with whatever you may be doing.

At the end of the day, pause to reflect upon and to give thanks for the insights and inspirations of this special day. Perhaps record some of your inspirations in a journal. Conclude your retreat with a final session of loving-kindness meditation (pp. 157–63).

Dedicate the positive energy and merit of the day's gifts as an ongoing source of inspiration in your own life, and as a wave of loving-kindness, inspiration, and blessings for those you love and for all beings.

▼▼ Our world is so crammed full with words, images, and sounds—our foremothers from centuries past would probably go batty if they were dropped off in 2002! And many of us are so focused on leaning into the future and doing the next thing that we can't stop and just BE. That's why it's critical that we cut everything off from time to time—that we unplug the phone, let the email pile up, and send the kids off to a friend's house. Our real power comes from knowing who we are and what we're here to do—and that begins with looking inside ourselves in silence. Solitude is part of the path to spiritual awareness.

Oprah Winfrey

2 STRATEGIES FOR
MASTERING STRESS ▼ ▼ ▼

ife's myriad changes often lead to an accumulation of stress. Here is a
compendium of simple, commonsense strategies for transforming mental
and physical tension into energy creatively and effectively expressed.
None of these strategies are new. Many will be familiar to you, but we often
need to be reminded. Circle the ones you'd like to remember more often.
Then add your own to the list:

TAKE TIME FOR YOURSELF

▼ Take time to be alone on a regular basis, to listen to your heart, check
your intentions, reevaluate your goals and your activities.
▼ Plan to do something each day that gives you energy, something you
love to do, something just for you.
▼ Take frequent relaxation breaks.
▼ Learn a variety of relaxation techniques and practice at least one
regularly.

FOCUS AND SIMPLIFY

▼ Simplify your life! Start eliminating the trivia.
▼ Practice consciously doing one thing at a time, keeping your mind

focused on the present. Do whatever you're doing more slowly, more intentionally, and with more awareness and respect.

CONNECT WITH OTHERS

▼ When you're concerned about something, talk it over with someone you trust, or write down your feelings.

▼ Create and maintain a personal support system—people with whom you can be "vulnerable."

▼ Seek out friends or professional help when you feel unable to cope.

▼ Practice stress-reducing communications: Clarify what you hear by paraphrasing ("I understand you to be saying... ") and active listening. Use "I want" instead of "I need," and "I choose to," rather than "I have to." Feel the difference in your mental attitude and your body when you do this.

STAY IN TOUCH WITH YOURSELF

▼ Say no when asked to do something you really don't want to do. Read a book on assertiveness if you have trouble doing this in a firm but kind way.

▼ Become more aware of the demands you place on yourself, your environment, and others to be different from how they are at any moment. Demands are tremendous sources of stress.

TAKE CARE OF YOUR BODY

▼ Exercise regularly!

▼ Monitor your intake of sugar, salt, caffeine, and alcohol.

▼ Take deep, slow breaths frequently, especially while on the phone, in the car, or waiting for something or someone. Use any opportunity to relax and revitalize yourself.

▼ Treat yourself to a massage or learn to massage your own neck, shoulders, and feet.

CONNECT WITH THE WORLD AROUND YOU

▼ Take time to be with nature, people, music, and children. Even in the city, noticing the seasonal changes of the sky or watching people's faces can bring about feelings of balance and harmony.

▼ Watch clouds or moving water. Notice the silence between sounds, the space between thoughts.

BE OPEN TO LEARNING ABOUT YOURSELF

▼ When you find yourself repeatedly angry in similar situations, ask yourself, "What can I learn from this?" Anyone or anything that can make you angry is showing you how you let yourself be controlled by expectations of how someone or something should be. When we accept others, ourselves, and situations for what they are, we become more effective in influencing them to change in the ways that we'd like them to.

▼ Use your own distress to teach yourself to be more patient, caring, and compassionate toward yourself and others.

▼ Choose not to waste your precious present life on guilt about the past or worry for the future.

STAY POSITIVE

▼ Carry a card with four or five personal affirmations written on it (for example, *I am calm and relaxed. I am confident and capable of handling any situations.*).

▼ Keep a positive, proactive attitude. As a wise sage once said, "If you can't do something about it, why worry? If you can do something about it, why worry?"

▼ Focus on what you *can* do.

TAKE CONTROL OF YOUR TIME

▼ Organize your life to include time for fun, spontaneity, and open spaces.

Set a realistic schedule allowing some transition time between activities. Eliminate unnecessary commitments.

▼ Learn to delegate responsibility.

▼ If your schedule is busy, prioritize your activities and do the most important ones first.

▼ Remember, it takes less energy to get an unpleasant task done right now than to worry about it all day.

NURTURE YOURSELF WITH JOYFUL ACTIVITIES

▼ Smile and laugh more.

▼ Remember to stop and smell the flowers.

3 GUIDELINES FOR CREATIVE VISUALIZATION ▼ ▼ ▼

Imagery and visualization are universal mental functions, common to every human being. Though they play a critical role in our psychological and physical health, performance, and creativity, these capabilities are poorly understood and are seldom developed to their full potential. By bringing these ordinarily unconscious mental processes into conscious awareness we can learn to dramatically expand the scope of possibilities available to us.

It is helpful to distinguish between spontaneous mental imagery and creative visualization. Imagery rich in information is continually arising within the mind—fantasies of the future, memories of the past, dreams, visions, our own self-image, and myriad expectations that we project upon our world. Properly understood, imagery is the stuff of revelation and intuition. Within the gestalt of a single mental image is enfolded information that—when unfolded into concepts, words, mathematical or musical formulas—may fill many volumes. Some mental images are experienced consciously, while others are edited by our belief system or are simply too subtle to be recognized.

While mindfulness of spontaneously arising mental imagery serves primarily a "readout" function, visualization is a more active, creative function of the mind. With visualization we are intentionally involved in generating and shaping the stream of mind-energy into prescribed mental images. Visualization equips us with a powerful tool for mentally simulating complex processes or possible futures that are beyond the scope of our ordinary perception and thinking. "Imagination is more important than knowledge," said Einstein, understanding the interdependence of creative vision and intuitive wisdom.

Understanding that every mental image directly influences our body, new dimensions of self-mastery or self-sabotage become clear to us. Although an actual or anticipated experience may last only a minute, our innate capacity to remember or anticipate the experience may trigger similar mental, emotional, and physiological reactions over and over again. Bringing these emotionally charged images to conscious awareness, we can then learn to creatively and productively control our imagination and not only master the psychosomatic symptoms associated with distress and anxiety, but also energize and strengthen positive qualities of mind. Learning the inner language of "listening" to mental imagery and "speaking" with creative visualization, we equip ourselves with critical skills for optimizing many of the functions of our mindbody and realizing extraordinary levels of health and performance.

For example, if we imagine that we are feeling the warm rays of the sun, this may trigger a response that dilates our blood vessels, warms our hands, and lowers our blood pressure. Images of aggression can lead to the secretion of neurotransmitters associated with anger or fear, increasing our heart rate, muscular tension, and blood pressure. Similarly, the image of biting into a tart, juicy grapefruit can cause saliva to flow; or the memory of a tender embrace may fill us with the pleasant tingles of sexual arousal.

By calling forth a memory of a peak experience we can awaken in the present moment those life-giving forces and strengths of character that inspired our performance in the past. Remembering the example of an inspiring teacher or role model, or visualizing their presence, can enable us to align our own thinking, will, and behavior with theirs.

The strategies listed below will help you discover and develop the imagery and visualization styles that work best for you.

PROJECTIVE AND ASSOCIATIVE VISUALIZATION

There are two approaches to visualization: projective and associative. Using projective visualization, you assume the view of an observer of the action— you will see yourself giving a dynamic presentation or skiing down a slope in deep powder snow. With an associative approach, you identify with the action and embody the experience—looking out through your mind's eye you behold the keen interest in the eyes of your listeners, or feel the spray of the snow in your face and sense an exhilarating thrill of aliveness. Each exercise that follows can be "viewed" from the detached objective stance of an outside observer, or as a vivid, virtual reality of affirmed embodied experience. Experiment and discover what works best for you.

REMEMBER, VISUALIZATION IS NOT ALWAYS VISUAL

Can you imagine hearing the tune "Jingle Bells"? How about smelling the smoke and feeling the warmth of a campfire? Visualization works best when you involve all of your senses to create a multisensory gestalt of synthetic experience.

THE KINESTHETIC, DIMENSIONAL, AND DYNAMIC APPROACH

In the space before you, visualize an object. Imagine what it would be like to reach out and touch that object. If you are visualizing an apple, reach out and hold it in your hand. Allow it to become real for you as you sense its shape, weight, and size. Imagine holding the hand of a loved one; sense its warmth and aliveness. Envision yourself flowing through a sequence of movements to accomplish a task; feel your body moving, carving out space with patterns of motion. Infuse your visualizations with a dynamic, radiant sense of energy and aliveness.

AFFIRMING THE IMAGE

Whether or not you can actually see or feel the visualized object or experience, mentally affirm that it is indeed there. This is like waking up one morning to find your surroundings shrouded in thick fog. Although you cannot see clearly the houses and trees around you, you will still know that they are there. If you are imagining an internal feeling, mentally and emotionally affirm that it is indeed a living reality within you, but at a level of sensitivity below the threshold of your awareness. With practice build the vividness of these qualities until you are confident that they are radiantly alive within you.

FILL IN THE DETAILS OR BEGIN WITH A FRAGMENT

You may find it helpful to begin with a sense of the outline of an object and to then fill in the details. For example, when visualizing a person, begin by envisioning her shape or form, and then mentally add the details as clearly as possible. Similarly, experiment by beginning with a tiny piece of the image, and then mentally develop it. Start by imagining a person's smile, then mentally paint in the rest of his face and body. Along the way, if portions seem to fade out or dissolve, gently focus the flow of imagery to bring those regions back into view.

AFFIRM THE COMPLETENESS OF THE IMAGE OR PROCESS

Although the total image or scenario may not appear to you clearly, affirm its completeness. If, for example, you are visualizing a healing process, imagine that it is worked through to completion. See, feel, and affirm yourself as healed and whole. Envision standing in the possibility as though it were an actual reality.

OBJECTLESS IMAGERY

Some of the most powerful types of visualization for enhancing health, performance, and understanding of the mind involve objectless imagery of volume, distance, and spatial relationships. Is it possible for you to imagine the volume of your hands, of your whole body? Sense the space and distance between you and the objects or people that surround you. Can you imagine hearing the silence before, between, and after sounds, or discovering the space between the thoughts and the images floating through your mind? As you become more intimately aware of space as a medium of relationship, connectedness, and communication, you discover that space connects everything–that separateness is a mere optical delusion of consciousness.

Beholding the dynamic, fluid, and insubstantial nature of mental images, you will be better prepared to work wisely with creative visualization. This insight into the fluid nature of mindstuff is of critical importance. Without this recognition, there is a danger of using visualization to further deepen the illusion of substantiality and solidity rather than to awaken greater wisdom, freedom, and power. Recognizing the dreamlike insubstantiality of the flow of images in the mind, and considering how compelled most people are by these largely unconscious images, a genuine sense of compassion may well up within you. Bringing the image-generating process of the mind into the domain of conscious awareness, compulsive reactivity will diminish, and your wisdom and freedom will grow. You will discover more creative options and make wiser decisions. Integrating these skills and insights, you will be well equipped to wisely use and apply these powerful visualization skills to enhance the creativity and quality of your life.

4 TRANSFORMING PAIN ▼ ▼ ▼

If a living system is suffering from ill health,
the remedy is to connect it with more of itself.
Francisco Varella

The Dalai Lama often reminds his students that the goal of the path of meditation is to fully awaken to our true nature and to become enlightened. To become enlightened, he has pointed out, we must perfect compassion, and to perfect compassion, we must encounter suffering. Taking this teaching to heart, a natural next reflection is that if this is really true, then what is the real meaning of pain or suffering in our lives and in our world?

Pain, suffering, loss, and dissatisfaction invite us onto a path of soul searching, self-reflection, and transformation. If instead of turning away or dulling our experience, we embrace and investigate it and allow it to open our hearts and minds to a deeper compassion and insight, there is great liberating potential in this. There are the sufferings of pain in the body manifesting as injury, disease, hunger, immobility, and dying. There are also the sufferings of mental anguish and disease of mind experienced as anxiety and fear, loneliness, confusion, or dissatisfaction that lead many people to look for skills to cope with, if not to master, their discomfort. There is also the suffering of the heart that has closed to itself out of guilt, blame, unworthiness, or shame, and has shut off from the world out of anger, jealousy, or fear. All of these conditions are painful and unsatisfactory. If our level of awareness is low, it takes more pain to get our attention. If we learn to pay attention to our minds, bodies, and relationships, the warning signs of pain will become apparent and can be dealt with when they are just whispers rather than screams.

Once recognized, our suffering may lead us to search for methods to heal the wounds in our bodies and minds, our hearts or spirits. Some methods distract us or take our attention elsewhere, effectively blocking our awareness of pain and often allowing conditions to worsen and further deteriorate. Other methods enable us to better understand the changing nature of our pain and to live more comfortably with the conditions in our bodies and in our lives that we associate with our suffering. Still other strategies are truly effective means of eradicating the causes of our suffering and putting an end to our mental and physical disease.

Traditionally, different meditation techniques have been used effectively to cope with or master pain. Though concentrative techniques can be effective at masking the pain, the emphasis of applying meditation to working with pain is that of directly investigating and understanding it. Upon careful examination of the field of sensations that we label "pain," we find that it is not a thing or unchanging entity. Rather pain is a nonentity, a dynamic field of sensations and feelings that changes with each moment and with each state of mind. The courage to face and understand our own suffering is the first step to working effectively with our own pain. It is also the first step in learning to open our hearts and minds enabling us to empathize and compassionately relate to the sufferings of others. By understanding our own wish to be free from our suffering, we begin to develop greater compassion, wishing that others might be free as well.

Over the years, we've worked with thousands of people in pain. Our unit at the hospital functioned as an unofficial pain clinic. Time after time we've worked with people in intractable pain due to injury, cancer, nerve damage, or fatal illness. From these people we've learned that the greatest suffering does not come from the torn or rotting flesh, or the tumor or the bedsores, but from their mental interpretation and response to the situation. Fear, helplessness, frustration, anger, guilt, and blame are clearly effective methods of intensifying the pain, constricting the body and mind to isolate, contract, and cut off that part of oneself from healing. Those who learn to open to pain, to investigate it and allow it to change, flow, and float freely in their bodies, take the first step toward mastering pain. Though this openness does not mean that the pain will go away, it does create a mental and emotional space in which pain is no longer related to as the enemy or as an emergency. With this openness we are able to accept, nurture, and love the part of us that is in pain. If we then bring the same quality of openness and reflection to our thoughts and emotional feelings, we will learn to recognize both the patterns of mind that intensify our suffering and the patterns of mind that bring greater harmony. In this way we become more responsible for optimizing our own self-healing potentials.

A further quantum leap in working with pain and suffering comes when we begin to use our own experience of pain as a means to open the heart in a caring and compassionate way to others. At this stage our self-centered fix-ation on our own suffering is transformed into a genuinely selfless outpour-ing of love, compassion, and caring that is mentally or even physically offered to others.

As we write this, the image of a man dying with AIDS comes to mind. He was a very spiritual man whose doctor had referred him to Joel to learn med-itation in order to better work with his extreme discomfort and to better face his impending death. At one of his visits, he described to Joel how during his sleepless hours throughout the day and night he would practice the heartfelt extension of love and compassion to others: the dying child down the hall, patients in all the hospitals in the vicinity, his family, and all oth-ers who were suffering as he was. Though isolated from most human con-tact, he found that reaching out to others in a sincere way somehow put his own pain in perspective, and his suffering diminished.

Approached with the right state of mind, many of the techniques in this book are effective means for working with physical and mental pain and for coming to a deeper sense of our own wholeness.

▼▼   Suffering is not enough.
       Life is both dreadful and wonderful.
       To practice meditation is to be in touch with both aspects.
       Smiling means that we are ourselves, that we have sovereignty
       over ourselves, that we are not drowned in forgetfulness.
       How can I smile when I am filled with so much sorrow?
       It is natural—
       you need to smile to your sorrow because you are more than
       your sorrow.
                                        —Thich Nhat Hanh

5 BALANCING BREATH, BRAIN, AND MIND ▼ ▼ ▼

Place a mirror up to your nose and breathe naturally. As you look at the two pools of condensation on the mirror you will notice that one is larger than the other. In fact, if you check throughout the day, you will notice that at any time you are breathing predominantly through one nostril or the other.

Every ninety minutes to two hours the dominant nostril changes; this will happen over a matter of minutes. For most people, the shift in dominance goes from right to left and back again roughly ten to twelve times every twenty-four hours. This cycle naturally alternating breathing has been known to inner science traditions for thousands of years, though it is only in the last decade that Western science has recognized and studied it.

We were once invited to advise a group of NASA researchers studying "Hazardous States of Awareness"—which referred to lapsing into drowsiness or falling asleep while flying a very fast and expensive aircraft on a long, boring flight. We were delighted and surprised to find that the primary brain mechanism they were studying was this connection between the quality of attention, the breath flow alternating between the two nostrils, and the rhythmic shift of dominance between the two hemispheres of the brain. The methods they were using included the nine-part breath from the concentration chapter (see pp. 64–65) and many of the principles presented in this section.

While current theories in neuroscience have greatly expanded upon and refuted many generalizations assumed in previous decades regarding the functions of the two hemispheres of the brain, some general principles still hold largely true. For example, activating the left hemisphere of the brain will generally augment our capacity to focus and gather high-resolution detailed information. Activating the right hemisphere, on the other hand, is generally associated with more diffuse qualities of attention that are more likely to lapse into drowsiness or sleep. Mental functions associated with spatial awareness, grasping a gestalt, or an intuitive sense of a situation are often associated with the right hemisphere. Mental functions of logical reasoning and language formulation are largely associated with the left hemisphere. Both ancient wisdom and modern research agree that the functions of either hemisphere of the brain are augmented and enhanced when you are breathing predominantly through the *opposite* nostril. For example, in moments when you fall asleep it is very likely that you will be breathing predominantly through your left nostril, and that the right hemisphere of your brain will be more active than the left. As breathing shifts from nostril to nostril, not only is there a shift in one's state of mind, but also in the fluctuations of neurotransmitters in the bloodstream and in nervous-system activity throughout the entire body.

Someday this understanding may provide modern science with valuable insight into the mechanisms and treatments of mental disorders. At a practical level, it may provide us with simple yet effective tools for shifting our brain-mind dominance toward the more logical and analytical mode of the left hemisphere or conversely toward the more intuitive or perceptual mode associated with right hemisphere function.

For thousands of years varieties of techniques have been used to optimize brain function by balancing the subtle energies of the mindbody. According to ancient traditions of meditation, the best time to meditate is when the breath flow is balanced between the two nostrils. This time of balance will occur in two ways: either naturally during the transition time between nostril dominance, when the energies of mind, brain, and body are most balanced, or when the meditator brings about this balance through techniques such as the one described below. In contemporary neurophysical terms, these times of balance would allow for an integration of rational and intuitive, detailed and global functions associated with the two hemispheres of the brain. At these times, information flows more smoothly across the corpus callosum, a bundle of brain fibers that forms the communications link between the two sides of the brain.

Understanding the breath-brain functions can not only enhance your meditation but can also be used to fine-tune your mindbody throughout the day. To do this, simply and frequently bring attention to your breath flow, your nostril dominance, and your predominant mode of mind. If you find it difficult to accomplish a particular task with your present state of mind-brain, try shifting your breathing pattern to the other hemisphere and mind style. To do this, first identify which nostril you are breathing through. Then inhale through the new nostril, exhaling through the previously dominant one for a few minutes until the breathing feels like it has shifted. This can be enhanced by visualizing the breath flow as clearing the nostrils and energizing the functions of the opposite brain hemisphere. It is especially useful to apply these techniques: (1) if you notice that your mind is dull, diffuse, or daydreamy when you need to accomplish a task requiring detailed precise attention, or (2) if you feel swept away by disruptive emotional feelings, agitation, or confusion. Since studies show that appetite and digestion are enhanced while we are in a right-nostril-dominant breathing cycle, you may choose to eat at times when this pattern occurs naturally, or even consciously shift this balance if you need to eat at another time. Similarly, most people will find that deep sleep is more quickly and easily achieved by lying on the right side, which shifts the breath dominance to the left nostril.

6 SPORTS: A WESTERN YOGA ▼ ▼ ▼

Sports, music, and dance each have something in common with meditative training. Each of these activities demands that we be fully present in what we are doing, yet at the same time maintain a suppleness and flow with the moment-to-moment changes of the process. The mental and physical discipline of sports or the performing arts trains the mind to access a wide range of concentrative and meditative states. The exhilaration of these activities is not just due to physical demands, but is also related to the naturally blissful, energized, creative, and peaceful experience of the quiet and concentrated mind.

Once we have successfully harnessed our wandering thoughts, new dimensions of awareness open up. Momentary peak experiences of being in the "flow state" with its effortless and extraordinary performance are quite common to athletes and artists. These moments of grace seem to happen spontaneously and are seldom fully understood or replicable, yet their memory lingers and our standards for what we know is possible may never be the same again.

The numerous examples of flow state or peak performance experiences reported by athletes and sports teams—though described by "jocks" rather than bearded sages—are strikingly similar to classical concentrative and meditative experiences.

Certainly not all of us have to dedicate our life to our sport, rather we can dedicate our sport to our life—approaching our training as a vehicle for honing those human qualities that enhance virtually all of the endeavors we set our minds to. There are countless men and women who have learned how to calm their minds through breath control, to transmute anger and fear into power, to let go as well as to hold on, to be sensitive and caring rather than callous. By learning to blend with inner and outer natural laws, many athletes have been able to tap reservoirs of extraordinary power, skill, and understanding, allowing them to perform in remarkable ways

▼▼ Sports training can develop an athlete's personality, improve physical and psychological skills, and lead one to discover unlimited possibilities of the human mind and body. Athletic performance is only a means to facilitate the athlete's self-actualization.

Tadeuz Rychta

The arena of athletic competition provides a laboratory in which mind-body skills can be tested and refined. Though the motivation may be different, the commitment and rigorous discipline of modern athletes is closely akin to practitioners of inner contemplative traditions. When faced with an equal in competition, one is forced to draw upon resources that are ordinarily considered beyond the range of one's capabilities. The orchestration of mental factors necessary to reach for this domain of extraordinary performance has catapulted many individuals and teams into realms of experience that are ordinarily the territory of yogis, mystics, and contemplatives.

This has resulted in a wave of interest that incorporates the conscious cultivation of mental fitness skills in conjunction with the practice of athletic and martial arts disciplines. On the field or on the mat, one receives moment-to-moment feedback on the interrelationship of mind and body. With practice one learns to minimize those mental and physical states that decrease and impair one's effectiveness, and to increase those that enhance one's performance.

Let us look at some examples of how these extraordinary states of mind can be developed and expressed in the arena of our life. The dynamic state of personal excellence in action has been examined in contemporary psychology at the University of Chicago by Mihaly Csikzentmihalyi, who has studied a broad range of intrinsically rewarding activities, all of which are marked by a similar experience, which he calls "the flow." The key elements of the flow are:

1. the merging of action and awareness in sustained, nondistractible concentration on the task at hand

2. the focusing of attention on a limited field of stimuli
3. self-forgetfulness with heightened awareness of function and body states related to the involving activity
4. skills adequate to meet the environmental demand
5. clarity regarding situation cues and appropriate responses

Flow states arise when there is an optimal correspondence between one's capability and the demands of the moment. The spectrum of the flow experience is bordered on the one hand by anxiety-inducing situations where demands exceed one's capability, and on the other by boredom, when one's capability far exceeds the demand.

A person in flow operates from a unified perspective. Their attention is completely absorbed in the activity without any dualistic sense of an "I" who is doing something. The moment this awareness is split and one becomes self-conscious, the flow state is interrupted.

Professional basketball player Patsy Neal tells us,

▼▼ There are moments of glory that go beyond the human expectation, beyond the physical and emotional ability of the individual. Something unexplainable takes over and breathes life into the known life. One stands on the threshold of miracles that one cannot create voluntarily. The power of the moment adds up to a certain amount of religion in the performance. Call it a state of grace, or an act of faith... or an act of God. It is there, and the impossible becomes possible.... The athlete goes beyond herself; she transcends the natural. She touches a piece of heaven and becomes the recipient of power from an unknown source.

The power goes beyond that which can be defined as physical or mental. The performance almost becomes a holy place—where a spiritual awakening seems to take place. The individual becomes swept up in the action around her—she almost floats through the performance, drawing on forces she has never previously been aware of.

A neurophysical interpretation of the significant characteristics of the flow state reveals that it requires both precision and fluidity in neurologic patterning, so that the brain can change in dynamic response to the fluctuating situational requirements. The flow state is not a static pattern of ongoing arousal, rather it demands flexibility. The chronically anxious or habitually aroused individual is likely to confront more situations in which his or her internal state is inappropriately tuned to environmental demands and is thus unable to access a flow state. Changing circumstances require changing internal states.

There are two ways of increasing the likelihood of flow experience: regulating environmental challenge to fit one's skills, as in games, or self-regulation of internal capacities to meet a greater variation in external demands. The disadvantage of the first is that flow remains situation bound, relying on a given set of environmental cues for its elicitation. Mental fitness disciplines such as relaxation, concentration, meditation would fulfill the latter strategy of producing a shift in internal state. Learning such skills maximizes the possibility for us to enter the flow state, while lessening the need to control the environment. Moreover, these approaches teach how to use a variety of self-tuning technologies that alter the basic process of mind, so that situations can be met from a flow state more frequently.

Epstein has recently suggested that one of the most rewarding aspects of long-distance running is what some have called the runner's high. She describes it as "drifting"...formerly known as "dreaming your life away." Epstein states:

▼▼ The standard by which I measure my run is not the degree to which I sweat or how fast a pace I set. It is not important to me whether I beat my own record or surpass my friends. Just give me a quiet, pleasant area to run and let me drift.

Epstein also noted that the evaluation of her runs was based on the amount of drifting she has been able to accomplish. It was acceptable occasionally to focus on some unusual or interesting sight, but speedy return to the state of drift was paramount.

One of the most celebrated descriptions of an experiential immersion in flow was given by ex–San Francisco quarterback John Brodie. In an interview with Michael Murphy, founder of Esalen Institute, Brodie described this extraordinary way of perceiving space and time:

▼▼ Often in the heat and excitement of a game, a player's perception and coordination will improve dramatically. At times, and with increasing frequency now, I experience a kind of clarity that I've never seen adequately described in a football story. Sometimes, for example, time seems to slow way down in an uncanny way, as if everyone were moving in slow motion. It seems as if I have all the time in the world to watch the receivers run their patterns, and yet I know the defensive line is coming at me just as fast as ever. I know perfectly well how hard and fast those guys are coming and yet the whole thing seems like a movie or a dance in slow motion. It's beautiful.

Descriptions by athletes of such events are abundant. These are common and are not purely the exclusive domain of the professional athlete. The time-defying total absorption of the backyard athlete or the runner's high of the professional marathon may be similar in origin. These experiences suggest that an alternative to the ordinary means of experiencing space and time lies within us all. Our challenge is to understand the mechanisms of these experiences and help people learn to consciously evoke these experiences rather than unconsciously stumble into them.

Lester Fehmi describes this state as "an unobstructed flowing of energy and experience through the mindbody system." He designed a method he called "open focus training" that works with spatial awareness and objectless imagery to decrease ordinary self-consciousness and the awareness of time and space. This state of integration he calls "no-time." He concludes that the way we attend affects all waking activity. Research on open focus and similar meditation techniques confirms that the disposition of attention, more than any other process of behavior that one can learn to control, directly governs one's state of mental and physiological well-being.

Explanation of the synchronous entrainment of a team is usually nebulous and vague. Yet theologian Michael Novak suggests that precise and coherent reorganization of individual and team resonance is demonstrated by these moments of team excellence:

▼▼ When a collection of individuals first jells as a team and truly begins to react as a five-headed or eleven-headed unit rather than as an aggregate of five or eleven individuals, you can almost hear the click;

a new kind of reality comes into existence at a new level of human development. A basketball team, for example, can click into and out of this reality many times during the same game; and each player, as well as the coach and the fans can detect the difference.

...for those who have participated in a team that has known the click of camaraderie, the experience is unforgettable, like that of having attained, for a while at least, a higher level of existence; existence as it ought to be.

With diligent practice and unwavering commitment, these extraordinary states of personal and team excellence can become the norm and not the fleeting exception. In an article entitled "The Liberal Arts and the Martial Arts" that appeared in the *New York Times*, Donald Levine described the stages of development that lead to the pinnacles of performance:

▼▼ One begins by self-consciously practicing a certain technique. One proceeds slowly, deliberately, reflectively; but one keeps on practicing until the technique becomes internalized and one is no longer self-conscious when executing it. After a set of techniques has been thoroughly internalized, one begins to grasp the principles behind them. And finally, when one has understood and internalized the basic principles, one no longer responds mechanically to a given attack, but begins to use the art creatively and in a manner whereby one's individual style and insights can find expression.

The fast-paced, colorful, and demanding nature of sports initially captures the interest of many people interested in testing the potential of their mind and body. With continued training, many athletes learn to equally value training time in the quiet depths of the mind as a domain of free play, self-healing, and regeneration, and as a source of strength and power to access new dimensions of performance. The continued melding of mental and physical technologies will empower athletes and teams of the future with the skills to far surpass the performance norms of today. With this contemporary approach to mental fitness training the best of both modern and ancient disciplines will be blended, enabling us to continually expand our understanding of what is possible for a human being or a team to accomplish.

7 CYBERPHYSIOLOGY AND BIOFEEDBACK: INNER TECHNOLOGIES OF MINDBODY AND SPIRIT ▼ ▼ ▼

The greatest thing in all education
is to make the nervous system our ally
instead of our enemy.

William James

Life is learning, and all learning depends on feedback. If we play an instrument, we listen to the quality of music and change the tuning accordingly. If we are cooking, we adjust the flavor of the food by tasting it. If we are doing target practice, we adjust our aim by watching the result of our shots. We continually rely upon feedback to refine our skills and reach our goals in any task, and the same is true with regard to living and working in relationships. By attending to the feedback of our bodies, our relationships, and our environment, we can learn, grow, and become more successful and effective in our lives.

Advances in modern medical technology are now making it possible to tune into the subtle changes of our own body by measuring, amplifying, and displaying this information to us. When this information is "fed back" to the individual whose biology is being measured, this process is called biofeedback training. When biofeedback training is combined with methods of relaxation, concentration, and meditation, this larger discipline is sometimes called *cyberphysiology*.

The disciplines of cyberphysiology and biofeedback are founded on thousands of years of experimentation, research, and refinement of teachings and skills. They demonstrate that the functions, actions, and capacities of our human body are profoundly influenced by mental images, emotions, attention, and intention. The modern epidemic of stress-related illnesses and extraordinary breakthroughs in human performance represent two ends of the spectrum of mental influence on our physical condition and abilities.

We are each born with the capacity to both enhance and undermine the quality of our health, yet most of us have never learned the basic inner skills for promoting our own health and well-being. Out of ignorance, many well-intentioned people mismanage their minds and create unnecessarily stressful and unhealthy conditions in their bodies. Yet, as people develop the inner skills of cyberphysiology, concentration, relaxation, meditation, and biofeedback, they learn how to focus their attention and their intention, and to organize their thoughts, emotions, and mental images in healthier ways. As a result, many physical ailments diminish in their frequency or intensity, or disappear altogether. As former clinicians running programs in medical centers, we have witnessed this a thousand times—often much to the amazement and inspiration of some of the more skeptical and less holistically oriented members of the medical staff.

To demonstrate the extraordinary potentials for intentional control of physiological systems, researchers Elmer and Alyce Green of the Menninger Foundation once invited an accomplished yogi, Swami Rama, to their psychophysiological control laboratory. The swami was wired to two temperature sensors so as to measure the change of blood flow to different parts of the palm of his hand. Under rigorous experimental conditions, the researchers watched as the swami demonstrated his ability to perform a medical miracle by consciously altering his circulation to make one part of his palm nearly seventeen degrees warmer than an area a couple of inches away. While the medical implications of such self-mastery were stunning and the researchers were very excited, it was sobering to hear Swami Rama say that it had taken him nearly twenty-five years to develop that level of self-control. A graduate student at Kansas State University who had heard about the experiment decided to see if he could learn the same control using thermal biofeedback training. Within two weeks of training with the equipment, he had achieved the same degree of extraordinary physiological control that the yogi admitted had taken him decades to learn.

Imagine the implications for modern medicine and science if many people were to learn to be aware of, control, self-regulate, and optimize their own body functions. Imagine what it would mean if the millions of people who needlessly suffer from stress-related illnesses were to learn the skills to consciously relax their tense muscles and reduce the symptoms of uptightness that they have stored in their digestive, circulatory, respiratory, and nervous systems. Imagine how different the quality of our lives and our world would be if many more people had the caring and discipline to learn these skills, refine their awareness, and awaken and develop the higher order capabilities of attention, compassion, creativity, wisdom, and intuitive intelligence that are rarely glimpsed, or fully matured, in a lifetime.

Biofeedback provides us with tools to accelerate our learning of mind-body fine-tuning. The key to this learning is assuming greater responsibility for our own health. As mentioned earlier, there are two strategies for recognizing disease. One is to allow the warning signs of imbalance to accumulate to the point of extreme discomfort or debilitation, and then to attempt to intercede with some radical or drastic intervention.

The alternative is to refine and intensify our internal awareness in order to recognize the initial subtle warning signs of disease and then to apply a simple remedy. As we learn to listen to the whispers of warning signs in our bodies and lives, we find there will be fewer screams of disease to have to deal with later.

Modern biofeedback technology is now enabling us to monitor and amplify many subtle signals from our bodies in order to bring information about ordinarily unnoticed and unconscious physiological processes to the level of conscious awareness. This revolution in modern science and medicine is an extension of our use of familiar technology. In many cases, similar or simplified versions of equipment that health care professionals have tested and measured us with are now being used to enable us to directly receive on-line biological information about our own body. Instead of an authority figure or expert interpreting the monitor readings and then treating us, we can gain greater self-awareness and control over our own internal process. In this way, we can experiment to find the subtle internal movement of mind that changes our body in the desired direction. As people learn these skills, they become measurably more self-empowered. This is often indicated on psychological tests that point to a shift from an "outer locus of control," where people feel victimized or less in control of their lives, to an "inner locus of control," where people are more confident and feel more able to make choices and be in control of their lives.

▼▼ Every change in the physiological state is accompanied by an appropriate change in the mental-emotional state, conscious or unconscious; and conversely, every change in the mental-emotional state, conscious or unconscious, is accompanied by an appropriate change in the physiological state...

Alyce and Elmer Green

Any method that helps us amplify the previously unconscious interplay of mental, emotional, and physiological processes enables us to learn how to change our lives for the better.

In practice it is almost as simple to use biofeedback to find out about our inner state of body as it is to use a mirror to find out about our outer appearance. What happens is that a passive sensor is attached over a site of muscle tension, blood flow, brain waves, or other physiological signal. The signal is then amplified and fed back to the person whose body it is coming from. Changes in the physiological state modulate the feedback signal that may be in the form of a tone that changes in frequency or loudness, a light bar or graph, a digital score, a computer game, video clip, or virtual reality display.

For example, if we were using a biofeedback instrument called an EMG (electromyograph), we would place a sensor over a tight muscle in a muscular region that is frequently tense. We would then use a monitor to amplify and feed back information about subtle increases and decreases of tension in order to quickly learn how to recognize and control the level of our tension or relaxation. In a similar way, one can learn to control hypertension, circulation, stress responses, or even to improve one's eyesight or enhance one's state of brain and mind. In the very near future, it is likely that enhanced sensors will provide us with moment-to-moment feedback on our blood chemistry and enable us to change our insulin levels or regulate the balance between hundreds of different neurotransmitters and hormones that regulate the functions of our body and states of mind.

▼▼ Each of us possesses everything that is necessary to explore our deepest nature.... No one else in all human kind can do it for us. The responsibility and opportunity for becoming aware of all that we most truly are and sharing it with others is ultimately our own.

Roger Walsh and Deane Shapiro

A contemporary revolution in health care is finding thousands of people actively involved in learning to control the diseases of modern times with psychophysical self-regulation training including meditation and biofeedback. The range of ailments being successfully treated in this way include hypertension, tension and migraine headaches, circulatory disorders, gastrointestinal disorders, chronic muscle tension, bruxism, and TMJ pain, chronic anxiety, compulsive addictions, and other stress-related symptoms.

Biofeedback is frequently used for teaching pain control and relaxation skills, enhancing neuromuscular coordination, speeding recovery time from illness, strokes, injury, and disease. Advanced applications of biofeedback training are helping people to increase the speed and accuracy of their senses, to accelerate their learning, and to turn on states of brain associated with mental calm, clarity, creativity, and intuitive intelligence.

As health care costs continue to climb, the practical sense and applications of biofeedback and the skills described in this book for helping people to optimize the workings of their own mindbodies will become increasingly important.

Most important, biofeedback is a tool for increasing our self-awareness and confidence in accepting greater responsibility to contribute to our own disease or well-being. Properly trained to interpret the myriad subtle messages our bodies are sending us, it is less likely that we will ignore the blatant warning whispers of accumulating stress and tension that unheeded may lead to life-threatening diseases.

Contrary to most medical treatments, with biofeedback training *you are the one in control.* With practice, most people quickly learn how to change their internal state for the better. Given the choice of energizing old harmful and self-abusive habits or not, a person learns an empowered option to go for the good.

Peak performance applications of biofeedback have attracted the attention of many of the world's finest athletes, performing artists, and creative minds who are interested in learning to reduce inefficient physical and mental patterns in order to train their bodies and brains for optimal performance. In pursuit of excellence, it is increasingly common for athletes, elite troops, and corporate executives to improve their health and performance by mentally rehearsing and refining their skills through the internal arts of meditation, visualization, and biofeedback-assisted training.

Biofeedback involves the development of four qualities of mind: attention, intention, creative visualization, and confidence.

Attention is the quality of mind that knows what we are attending to. To the degree that we can keep our attention on what we are doing, we can say that our attention is concentrated and stable.

Intention is the capacity that enables us to mentally direct our attention and action toward accomplishing our goals.

Creative visualization is the primary control language that enables us to mentally direct our attention and action toward accomplishing our goals.

Confidence or faith naturally emerges through the successful application of the prior three qualities. Fueled by our heightened self-esteem, our self-mastery skills continue to develop.

The misalignment of these factors allows our subconscious fears and anxieties to become physically manifested as disease, debilitation, or a vulnerability to accidents. Properly orchestrated and consciously directed, the power of our attention, intention, and imagery synergize to enable us to realize our capacity for extraordinary levels of health and performance.

We've been asked if biofeedback is "electronic Zen." Well, biofeedback software and hardware cannot do the learning for you, but using them can help you accelerate your learning to distinguish the mental states and attitudes that lead you toward or away from the physiological states of health or peak performance. Especially when it comes to developing the refined qualities of attention that are cultivated in meditation, neurofeedback—a type of "brain wave" or EEG biofeedback—can be very helpful. One day we were showing Chagdud Rinpoche, a respected Tibetan doctor and accomplished meditator, how biofeedback training worked, when he exclaimed:

"Ah! This is just like meditation. When I try to meditate it doesn't work. But when I meditate, it works!"

Regardless of the discipline, whether relaxation, concentration, meditation, or biofeedback, maximizing effort will never optimize your mindbody control. In fact, the state of mind most successful in directing our body to change for the better is classically referred to as "passive volition," "voluntary surrender," or "doing without trying." This quality of mind is best tuned in to by having a clear intention and image of the desired state of mindbody and then simply allowing it to happen effortlessly. The biofeedback process itself will let you know when you are on the right track and when you are trying too hard.

To get a picture of this key to self-mastery, an image comes to mind from the "biocybernautic training" we designed for the U.S. Army Green Berets' Jedi Warrior Training Program. Imagine a group of Special Forces troops each connected to biofeedback devices that were connected to toy racecars. The more they relax, the faster their car goes. Imagine them competing to see who can win the race by relaxing the most and the quickest. The pressure is on, and guess what—the harder they try to relax or to win, the quicker they lose control and their car stops dead in its tracks.

Biofeedback training opens new dimensions of power and self-mastery for tough "can-do guys" who are used to being in control on the outside, but who may actually be quite out of control on the inside—which leaves them vulnerable when the pressures and complexities of their lives increase. It makes it clear that the inner game of true self-mastery is ultimately less about effort and more about learning the exquisitely subtle balance of intention combined with a receptive quality of mindful attention. *Trying* to relax in an effortful way will never lead to success. In practical application this means that once you master these skills, then even in the midst of extreme intensity you will be more optimally tuned, present, sensitive to change, adaptable, intuitively responsive, and more likely to recognize options, make wiser choices, and create the best outcomes in difficult situations.

In the near future, revolutions in education will hopefully prioritize biofeedback and self-regulation training as a foundational discipline in grade schools—just like reading, writing, and arithmetic encourage a new generation of children to grow up with an attitude of greater confidence, self-empowerment, and responsibility for their own well-being. Especially for children growing up in circumstances that might leave them feeling disempowered, developing these skills could make a world of difference.

As technology advances and the stresses of our modern world continue to accelerate, interest in cyberphysiology and biofeedback could find many people learning to master their own stress and enhance their performance. Instead of watching TV or surfing the Internet, attention could be devoted to personal development using digitally enhanced contemplations assisted by multimedia computer biofeedback games with incredibly compelling graphics and scenarios.

Creativity and microcircuitry are currently being combined to develop a future generation of computer games in which the winners will be the men or women with the greatest mindbody self-mastery. Couples could learn to synchronize their heartbeats or brain waves and come into a more intimate attunement to one another. Parents and children could play cyberphysiology games that help them deepen their connections with themselves and each other. Cyberphysiology and biofeedback games will introduce us to new dimensions of personal mastery, learning, competition, and cooperation. Here winning would be determined by whoever can relax the most under pressure, or the goal may be to deeply relax but remain alert, or to synchronize one's heart beats or brain waves with one's challenger.

On the noetic frontier, the decades to come will witness further advancements in technology and research in human consciousness. As software and hardware continue to become more sophisticated, and our capacity to measure and feed back information regarding very subtle changes in bioelectromagnetic fields increases, the quantum effects of the mind on matter will become inspiringly apparent. Though our minds are continually affecting our own physiological state, the profundity of these effects has only been known by practitioners of contemplative disciplines prior to the advent of modern biofeedback and medical monitoring technology. As we continue to refine our technology and our attention, we will surely discover what inner scientists and meditators have known through direct intuitive experience for millennia—that matter, be it a body or a world, is intimately pervaded by and responsive to the mind.

Recent research at Princeton University's Engineering Anomalies Research Project, at Menninger Foundation, at Stanford University, and at numerous other prestigious institutions worldwide has already begun to investigate and document the impact of conscious, focused intention on various quantifiably measured external things, such as computer functions.

Continued breakthroughs in technology will herald a renaissance of research into the nature of human consciousness as we witness the undeniable effect that mental intention can have on microtechnology—technology that is at the heart of the greatest sources of creative and destructive power in our world. Since these tools have been demonstrated to be subject to the power of our individual and collective intention, we will hopefully come to recognize that understanding these extraordinary human capacities is vital to our future development.

Thousands of well-controlled scientific studies on prayer, and on "non-local effects" of the mind consistently demonstrate that the same qualities of mind—attention and intention—that enable us to create changes in our own bodies, if properly directed, can make measurable changes beyond our bodies. The growing evidence is profoundly compelling, and the data suggests that even ordinary, untrained people have the latent ability to develop and demonstrate extraordinary abilities, many of which challenge our cherished "mental models" and assumptions regarding the nature of mind and reality. This trend in research is rapidly and radically expanding the dimensions of scientific inquiry and challenging researchers to become ever more adept in both the inner and outer sciences.

Regarding the relationship between extraordinary events, the nature of the mind, and biofeedback, one of the great pioneers of biofeedback research, Barbara Brown, has said:

▼▼ If mental activity truly originates from our brain cells, then it is logical to assume that psychic phenomena also use these same brain cells. We assume this because psychic activity involves a change in mental activity; otherwise, it could not be integrated, stored, recalled, and communicated by human means. Telepathic information must have entry into the universe of the brain cells where the "picture" of the information is developed. Even if the psychic information gets into the brain supernaturally, it must go through the ordinary channels of brain processing to get out of the brain to be communicated to other people. This means that there is a brain physiological impression of the psychic experience. If that impression is there, then we should be able to find it. If biofeedback can be used with this brain indicator to bring psychic abilities under voluntary, predictable control, this will be one of the most explosive discoveries that biofeedback can make.

As research into the nature of human creativity, health, and peak performance provides us with a clearer image of what is possible for a human being, biofeedback and cyberphysiology training will provide us with a powerful, effective, and entertaining means for strengthening those psychophysical latencies within us that will open new dimensions of health, creativity, love, understanding, extraordinary performance, and appreciation for the preciousness and potentials of our lives.

▼▼ I have no doubt whatever that most people live, whether physically, intellectually, or morally, in a very restricted circle of their potential being. They make use of a very small portion of their possible consciousness...much like a man who, out of his whole bodily organism should get into a habit of using and moving only his little finger.... We all have reservoirs of life to draw upon, of which we do not dream.

William James

PART FIVE

▼ ▼ ▼ **MEDITATION IN THE WORLD OF WORK**

The key to our inner resources is self-knowledge.
Self-knowledge is gained by personal development—that is,
by collecting experiences out of which new insights
and wisdom are born.... This comes close to being the
meaning of life. Consequently the raison d'être for a
company is to supply an environment in which the personal
development of human beings involved in the company
can best take place.... What a precious gift to humanity and
our planet it would be if the remarkable knowledge we
have achieved should be united with wisdom. Then our
planet would be the paradise it is meant to be. Business
life has the opportunity to bring that gift forward.

Rolf Osterber

1 RELAXATION, CONCENTRATION, AND MEDITATION AT WORK: AN INSPIRING EXAMPLE ▼ ▼ ▼

The following story offers a glimpse of one of the many ways that concentration and meditation might offer focus and inspiration within a business or work setting.

The crimson sunrise over the Canadian Rockies sets the maple trees ablaze in a glory of autumn colors. Silently we sit together. Leaders and corporate change champions, mostly engineers—all are members of the Change Strategy teams from seven leading companies: four major oil companies, one large utility corporation, an international construction company, and a university hospital. Linking us are many shared concerns, aspirations, and challenges.

We are gathered here as the crew for a "Corporate Learning Expedition," sponsored by ICOD, the International Center for Organization Design, for which we are core faculty members. Our mission is to support each other in designing the most sustainable and successful organization for each company to meet the challenges of the next ten years. Over the course of the next year, we will meet together for four retreats, to share our knowledge and experience, and to support each team in formulating its most viable and sustainable organization design to meet the challenges of the decade ahead.

At the end of last evening's opening session, a leader from one of the four oil companies suggested that we set a time and place for some "focusing and centering" at the beginning of our intense and busy days. "Let's get together in the Glacier Vista Lounge at 7 A.M.," he said to the fifty expedition members. "Everyone is welcome and I've asked Joel and Michelle Levey to help us get focused with some coaching tips from their meditation and personal mastery training for the Green Berets, Olympic athletes, and other businesses like ours. I don't know about you, but I can use all the help I can get to keep my energy high on these long days where the stakes are high and the pressure is on. If you are interested, set your clock and join us in the morning."

As 7 A.M. approached we walked across the campus of the Banff Center toward our meeting room. Around a corner we overheard a couple of engineers as they walked ahead of us. "I've read about this personal mastery stuff, but I've never really done anything like this before," said one. His buddy nodded and replied, "Yeah, me too. But look, if they did this kind of work with guys in Special Ops and with Olympic athletes, it can't be too New Age. You know me, if it works, I'll use it. Who knows, maybe I'll pick up a few ideas to improve my golf game!"

We settled into the room just as the first rays of dawn ignited the maple tree outside into a blaze of autumn colors. By 7 A.M. nearly a third of the whole team had arrived. Most of them had never done anything like this before, especially at work, and the air was charged with a sense of curiosity and self-consciousness. "Amazing" said our sponsor looking around with surprise and delight. "I thought we'd only have a handful of people. Look at all of us here." At the request of the group, we offered a few simple suggestions to help people organize and focus their attention in preparation for the work to come. We explained that we'd take a three-phase approach: first a few minutes to create context, then some brief instruction followed by fifteen minutes to practice, and finally some time to share insights or ask questions before breakfast.

To create context we pointed out the value of doing the inner work necessary to improve the quality of our outer work. We introduced the notion that "control follows awareness" and explained that we can only manage what we are mindful of. We discussed the performance advantages of being mindful by contrasting it to mindlessness. When we are mindless, we noted, we lapse into reactivity; habit rules, and it is impossible to be creative. Finally, we explained how our capacity for complex and creative systems-thinking is directly proportionate to our development of the quiet mind skills that determine the quality of our attention.

"If you are like most people, you have already mastered mindlessness and distraction. This morning we would like to introduce you to some new skills and challenge you to learn how to be wholeheartedly present or mindful, focused here and now in the present moment. Upon reflection you will notice that this moment has two important characteristics. First, it is the only place that you have any leverage to create change in your life or work. Second, it is elusive, fleeting, and constantly changing. Recognizing this, you will understand that mindfulness represents a flow or continuity of attention. Our challenge is to build this continuity of mindfulness by learning how to catch the wave-form of awareness and ride it without falling off into mindlessness or distraction."

"With this in mind, let's learn how to develop our mindfulness." Having created some context for *why* to train, we offered a few guidelines for *how* to train. We suggested that people begin by focusing their intention or motivation. We explained that one of the first steps in focusing the mind is to be clear on intention. Knowing what is important to us can help to stabilize and focus the mind. To do this, we invited everyone to bring to mind the circle of "stakeholders" who would be influenced by their decisions: their coworkers and loved ones supporting them back home; their suppliers and customers spread all over the globe; the members of their local and regional communities who would be influenced by their work; and the generations to come who would live with the impact of their decisions.

Building on the clarity of intention, we invited people to begin to build the power of their mindfulness by focusing their attention on the natural flow of their breath. "As you inhale, simply know that you are breathing in. As you exhale simply know that you are breathing out. As you breathe, begin to collect all your wandering thoughts and gather your loose ends to arrive fully focused right here and now. As you use your breathing to help you get focused, stay relaxed. If you have a tendency to try too hard, one strategy to keep from taking yourself too seriously is to hold a sort of half smile to yourself inwardly as you enjoy your breathing. Use some discipline to keep your mind on what you are doing, so that when the time comes, you'll be better able to keep your mind on your work. As you are mindful of your breathing, be attentive to the emergence of distracting thoughts. If or when your attention wanders off, notice if it is drawn to a fantasy of the future or to a memory of the past. Make a mental note of the distraction, and then as you inhale, simply draw your attention back to focus mindfully on what you are doing, being mindful of your breathing."

To help those who were particularly distracted by the chatter of their internal dialogue, we suggested that they experiment with synchronizing their breathing with the quiet mental repetition of two words. We explained that since the mind is busy thinking or talking to itself most of the time, using a quiet mental recitation is an effective strategy to harness and focus mental activity in a more intentional and productive way. With each inhalation we suggested making a brief mental note, "Arriving..." and breathing out the mental note, "Home...." "Arriving...home.... Arriving...home...." As an alternative, we suggested that people could also experiment with, "Here...now.... Here...now...."

Having created some context and offered some simple instruction, we suggested that people simply stay with this mindful breathing practice for about ten minutes in order to quiet, calm, and focus their minds.

After ten minutes, we suggested that each person turn their attention to quietly thinking deeply and clearly about the work and strategic challenges of the day. We offered a reminder that if the mind wandered to unrelated thoughts people be mindful of the distraction and use discipline to return the focus of their thoughts to the subject they had chosen. At the end of these fifteen deep and quiet minutes, we invited the group to debrief and to discuss their insights and inspirations about how their inner work had informed their outer work.

One of the engineers in charge of a new refinery commented, "I've done this kind of mental fitness training on my own for years, but never with a group of people that I work with. I've always wondered how it would be to work with a group of people who knew how to get focused and work in a more focused mind state together."

The foreman of a new drilling site observed, "I never knew that my mind could get so clear and quiet in such a short time. This is like learning how to push the *clear* button on my mental calculator. I never realized how learning to clear the slate could help me think more deeply and clearly. Thanks, coach!"

One of the senior vice presidents added, "You know, I think my greatest learning from this morning is that other people that I work with are interested in this inner work too!" People nodded. Looking around, his gaze met the eyes of people whom he worked with on a daily basis and people he had known for years from the other oil companies.

A plant manager for another drilling operation reflected aloud, "I coach rugby and I've worked with some of these mental focusing techniques for years. What we did this morning was real affirming of what I've sort of learned from the inside out. Thanks a lot."

Then, the director of human resources for another company spoke up: "I've been interested in this mind fitness work for years and I've sort of dabbled in it a bit. It's really great to have others that I work with engaged in this inquiry. Just imagine if we were to begin our working sessions back at the office with some quiet time like this to get focused and collect our thoughts. It's inspiring to see how clear, calm, and focused my thinking can be after such a short time. If we could do more of this work on an ongoing basis, we'd really be an unbeatable team!"

"My doctor's been telling me I've got to learn how to relax and let go of my stress or I'm going to have another heart attack," said one of Information Technologies' VPs. "I always thought this stuff was kind of strange, but you know this mindfulness of my breathing gives me a sense of myself like what I touch when I'm out fishing on a warm spring day. If I work at it, I bet I could tap into this sense of presence, clarity, and calm whenever I want. Wait till I tell my doc—will he ever be surprised." At that point someone laughed and chimed in, "Okay, it's time to break this huddle and get to work. We've got forty-five minutes before the whole team circles up. Who's ready for a cup of coffee and some breakfast?"

For the days that followed we continued to meet in the mornings before breakfast. Each day the circle grew as more of the team joined us. Some of the others who preferred to run, walk, or sleep in made a point to join us for breakfast, where the conversation tended to focus a lot on how the quality of mind is related to the quality of life and work. Questions about finding more balance between personal and professional lives, and on how to improve one's golf game were common. For some, these quiet morning sessions provided a deep sense of communion and connection with themselves, their team, their natural surroundings, and what was most essential or sacred in their lives.

After one of the strategic planning meetings with the staff, some of the leaders who hadn't been attending the morning sessions invited me to lunch. They started talking about how the energy level and performance of the whole team had bumped up a notch since the morning focusing sessions had begun. As one of the senior VPs put it, "You know, the members of our team who've been attending your morning sessions have really made some significant contributions to the breakthroughs that our team has had. I'm not sure what you've been doing in your morning sessions, but we'd like to encourage you to keep up the good work! We need all the inspiration and clear thinking we can get on our team if we're going to meet our goals, and this inner work seems to be making a real difference."

Over the months to come, this momentum continued and took different forms among the different company teams. When we flew in to Calgary to do some strategic work with one of the teams a month later, the director of operations gave us a call at the hotel, "Welcome back! Say, I forgot to tell you two to plan on showing up forty-five minutes before our meetings start while you are here. Some of us have taken over the boardroom in the mornings to do some focusing work before work. Not everyone comes, but for those of us who do, it has made a big difference. Some of us have some questions and want to see if we can bump our personal mastery work up a notch while you are in town. Will you come and join us?" We smiled and said to him, "You've got a deal, we'll meet you at your office at 6:55 in the morning."

The next morning we sat quietly in the boardroom on the twenty-seventh floor. In the predawn light the ghostly pillars of steam rose in a gray sky above the silent skyscrapers in this tiny corner of the frozen Alberta plains. For a moment, we're back in jeans at Glacier Vista with the maple tree ablaze in the crisp crimson dawn. *Arriving...home...here...now....* Sitting here quietly with these friends and fellow explorers, we smile to each other with the joy of beginning another precious day of life, and work, in such a special way.

2 LEADERSHIP AND SPIRIT AT WORK ▼ ▼ ▼

Without a global revolution in the sphere of human consciousness, nothing will change for the better in the sphere of our being as humans.... The salvation of this human world lies nowhere else than in the human heart, in the human power to reflect, in human meekness and in human responsibility.

Václav Havel

I n our own work we are often invited to help revitalize the health and spirit of leaders, teams, and large organizations around the globe. Working internationally we have the opportunity to work closely with people from many countries, professions, and many spiritual and philosophical traditions. Again and again we find a universal interest—if not yearning—in finding a way of living and working that is less depleting and more life affirming, one that encourages greater health and meaningful connectedness to a larger, more universal whole.

It seems that the dizzying complexity and breakneck pace of our modern lives have exiled many of us from the vitality of our authentic nature. We have lost sight of what our ancestors saw as essential—the importance of family, creative expression, heartfulness, and a deep, spiritual connectedness with our world and the living creatures who share it with us. There is an emptiness in many people's lives and an uneasy feeling that something vital has been lost, yet often we don't even remember what it was. One woman executive, attending an off-site seminar with one of our colleagues, expressed such a sentiment in a poignant poem that she wrote during the session: "Ten years ago I turned my face for a moment, and it became my life." For some of us, it feels like something essential in our lives is calling us home, though we don't even know what to call it. In the classical literature it is said that the greatest obstacles to discovering the presence of the sacred reality of life are a lack of mindfulness, confidence, faith, or discipline. With this in mind, the following anecdotes from the world of work are offered with the wish that they may inspire you and remind you that whether we recognize it or not, something deep, sacred, and soulful is alive, well, and attempting to emerge more fully through our lives, work, and organizations.

IN SEARCH OF WHOLENESS

▼▼ The most exciting breakthrough of the 21st century will occur not because of technology, but because of an expanding concept of what it means to be human.

John Naisbitt

We often hear people say that their wholeness as a human being is not welcome at work, and they are expected to leave their values, feelings, and physical needs at home. These comments are as common from executives as from blue-collar workers. To ignore or deny any of our many dimensions is foolish, dangerous, and unfortunately quite common, especially in the institutions of our workaday world. What we ignore or disown we tend to waste or destroy.

Most dis-ease, be it physiological, sociological, or ecological, begins with "whispered" warning signs. Only if these are ignored do we find ourselves in trouble, as the whispers become "screams." Ignorance is the root of most dis-ease. We are at a time when our ignorance has compromised the integrity of our ecosystem, when our social structures and families are collapsing, and when, in America, we are paying more than $1.3 trillion each year for disease care. This is more than the combined annual profits of all of the Fortune 500 companies, and business pays more than 40 percent of the bill. Yet some leading medical researchers believe that as much as 95 percent of all illness is due to our unwise choices and mismanagement of our minds, bodies, and lifestyle habits.

As complex, multi-dimensional, living beings, we are endowed with miraculous capacities for sensory discovery of our world, creative physical movement and communication, a broad spectrum of emotions, an inconceivable capability for creative imagination, intelligence, and thinking, and a nervous system with an extraordinary ability for intuitive discernment of our world at a far greater breadth and depth than mere thinking or ordinary perception can ascertain.

At our heart and core, inseparable from the rest, is a quality of radiant and receptive presence, a creative and compassionate intelligence that defies description. In the English, we may name this "consciousness," in the psychological sense, or "spirit," the animating force within all things, if we take a more sacred view.

Paradoxically, this illusive dimension of our deepest being is at the heart of our humanity, and being universal in proportions, it transcends the narrow confines of our personal identity. While spirituality and religion are related, they are often confused. The following classic words from Rachel Naomi Remen, M.D., offer a profound insight into this important relationship.

▼▼ The most important thing in defining spirit is the recognition that spirit is an essential need of human nature. There is something in all of us that seeks the spiritual. This yearning varies in strength from person to person, but it is always there in everyone.... Spiritual is not the religious. A religion is a dogma, a set of beliefs about the spiritual and a set of practices which arise out of those beliefs. There are many religions and they tend to be mutually exclusive. Every religion tends to think that it has "dibs" on the spiritual—that it's "The Way." Yet the spiritual is inclusive. It is the deepest sense of belonging and participation. We all participate in the spiritual at all times, whether we know it or not. There's no place to go to be separated from the spiritual, so perhaps one might say that the spiritual is that realm of human experience which religion attempts to connect us to through dogma and practice. Sometimes it succeeds and sometimes it fails. Religion is a bridge to the spiritual—but the spiritual lies beyond religion. Unfortunately in seeking the spiritual we may become attached to the bridge rather than crossing over it.

To say that there is no place for spirit, or consciousness, in our business and organizational life is as foolish as saying there is no place for our bodies and minds at work. Let's embrace reality. We are multidimensional human beings, and business, as all other arenas of human activity, will be handicapped without drawing inspiration from the full spectrum of our humanity.

THE INNERWORK OF INSPIRED LEADERSHIP

▼▼ A leader is a person who must take special responsibility for what's going on inside him or her self, inside his or her consciousness, lest the act of leadership create more harm than good. The problem is that people rise to leadership in our society by a tendency towards extroversion, which means a tendency to ignore what is going on inside themselves. Leaders rise to power in our society by operating very competently and effectively in the external world, sometimes at the cost of internal awareness. I've looked at some training programs for leaders. I'm discouraged by how often they focus on the development of skills to manipulate the external world rather than the skills necessary to go inward and make the inner journey.

Parker Palmer

Most often we are invited to work with an organization by a spirited leader. These people are generally the innovators and altruists in their organizations who really care about people and are committed to building a team or organization that brings out the best in them. Often these leaders express a spiritual yearning, though they aren't necessarily particularly religious. They are willing to think deeply, take risks, and act to get what they want for others.

▼▼ As we are coming to understand, spiritual values in leadership are not a passing trend but the integration of a new level of awareness that will enhance community in the workplace.

Barbara Krumsiek, President and CEO, Calvert Group, Ltd.

Dr. Stephen E. Jacobsen, a former business entrepreneur and now ordained minister, observed that though leaders in business had a difficult time clearly defining "spirituality," they did believe and speak strongly about its importance in forming the values, ethics, and beliefs that they bring to work. This diverse group of business leaders of different genders, backgrounds, organizational settings, and locations shared a common belief that spirituality is at the heart of their business activity. They regarded "spirituality" as a means of integrating self and the world, and affirmed that life is a seamless whole system with an absence of boundaries between what is "spiritual" and what is "secular."

Spirited leaders live with deep questions, often catalyzed by major breakdowns or breakthroughs in their life. Their heartbreaks, heart attacks, or near-to-death experiences expanded their consciousness and offered glimpses of a larger, sacred reality. Many have fought for their freedom or health, others for human rights, or for sobriety, and are willing to take a strong stand to help others. They are often people of strong faith and determination, whose personal epiphanies and tragedies have cracked open their hearts and souls to the sacred presence and grace at the heart of humanity. As a result, their life is dedicated to helping others discover their own potential, and their work becomes a vehicle to fulfill this purpose. Having hit the wall and broken through, they are willing to take risks and create opportunities for their people to work in ways that affirm and respect the integrity of their health, dignity, and spiritual wholeness.

▼▼ The first act of a great leader, I believe, is an act of faith.
It's believing that human nature is the blessing, not the problem.
Meg Wheatley

Suzanne, the VP of information systems for one of America's oldest and largest financial institutions, is an inspiring example of such a leader. Shortly after she returned to work after a close encounter with a life-threatening illness, the senior VP of her division launched a new "Vision and Mission Statement." It called for a radically different approach to achieving world-class information technology by developing a culture of high-performance teamwork, effective change management, and continuous learning. His team of 3,500 were told that the challenge would require "each and every one of you to become a bit of a visionary to make this Vision a reality.... I'm not smart enough to do this all by myself, so I need all of you to take some ownership for bringing this Vision alive."

In her search for a way to help her team meet this challenge, someone gave Suzanne an article on our work and she called to talk with us about how we might support her team. Talking with her we learned about her struggle to regain her health and her concern that others faced with the increasing work stress might experience similar threats to their own health. She wanted to offer a program to help them "take better care of themselves and support each other more effectively at work." Working with Suzanne, we designed a pilot program for her teams that emphasized a synergy of personal, team, and organizational development. The success of this pioneering project quickly ignited interest for similar programs in many other departments.

Bill, a former Catholic priest on Suzanne's team, offered the following explanation for the success of the program: "The principles we are applying, when understood and taken together, give us a picture of a new way we can live and work. It's an inside-out approach to change. If managers ask: 'How do we get our work done more efficiently, with a better end product?' I'd tell them that, along with improving the work process, go out and build trust, communicate honestly, support each team member, and find ways to drive out the fear and relearn the idea that it's important for everyone to seek balance and wholeness in and through our work. When this catches fire, an epidemic of sanity—even love—can spread."

"We've made some big strides towards making the Vision a reality in this year," said Suzanne. "But our people know this is really a journey of self-discovery that we are on, and that it never really ends. Our work here is to learn about constantly renewing ourselves, our team, and renewing our organization—one day at a time."

SPIRIT AND SYSTEMS THINKING

▼▼ My own working assumption is that we are here as local Universe information gatherers. We are given access to the divine design principles so that from them we can invent the tools that qualify us as problem solvers in support of the integrity of an eternally regenerative Universe.

R. Buckminster Fuller

At the heart of both business success and spiritual inquiry is the ability to think about and perceive our world in terms of dynamic, complex, whole systems. Both a systems view and a spiritual view of life and work invite a contemplation of profound interrelatedness across potentially limitless dimensions. For both disciplines, fruition is realized by discovering and applying our insights in ways that enable us to improve the quality of our lives and the overall health of the whole system.

When applied to understanding our place in the universe, systems thinking reveals an ever expanding and awe-inspiring panorama of complex and multidimensional interrelationships that span the farthest reaches of space-time and weave all living beings into a web of profound interdependence within a seamless wholeness. Again, we return to Einstein's words:

▼▼ A human being is part of the whole called by us universe, a part limited in time and space. We experience ourselves, our thoughts and our feelings as something separate from the rest. A kind of optical delusion of consciousness. This delusion is a kind of prison for us, restricting us to our personal desires and to affection for a few persons nearest us. Our task must be to free ourselves from this prison by widening our circle of compassion to embrace all living creatures and the whole of nature in its beauty.... We shall require a substantially new manner of thinking if mankind is to survive.

One of the most effective ways to hone our systems thinking and to develop a spiritual outlook on our life-work is to view ourselves as embedded within this vast network of interrelationships. In this vast network, there is only one of you, and there are billions of others who share similar core aspirations. Likewise, your business or organization is one of millions in a world desperately in need of help. Keeping in mind that over the course of your lifetime, countless people might be influenced by your work, ask yourself: If you were to live your life well and in a way that would bring you the greatest satisfaction and fulfillment, would you focus more on your own personal gratification or on helping others?

▼▼ The only ones among you who will be truly happy

are those who have sought and found how to serve.
Albert Schweitzer

A common meeting ground for systems thinking, consciousness development, and spiritual practice lies in the quality of our intentions. The spiritual potency of our actions is said to be determined by considering:

▼ Is it good for all of our stakeholders, i.e., for "all my relations"?
▼ Will the impact bring lasting benefit in a sustainable way, e.g., "unto the seventh generation"?

With the proper motivation and presence of mind, any action can become an act of devotion or an expression of spiritual concern and development. For example, as you read this chapter, can you imagine yourself sitting here at the center of your universe? Surrounding you are all your loved ones, family, and friends, and all your coworkers, customers, suppliers, and stakeholders in your work—everyone whose efforts in some way enrich or influence your life, and all those whom you influence directly or indirectly by your actions. Here are the members of your carpool, circles, support groups, classes, clubs, religious community, little league, soccer or basketball teams.... All living beings are here. And all your ancestors, and the generations to come who will live with the impact of your decisions and actions, are also here surrounding you.

Now consider if you, by reading and taking to heart this chapter or this book, or by doing your work today, are inspired by an insight that enables you to become a more wise, kind, and inspiring human being, and if you were to live in a way that was helpful to others, how many people's lives might you impact, directly or indirectly, over the course of the next year? Or, over the course of your lifetime? Remember, if you touch the heart of another human being, you change them forever!

Reflecting in this fashion for a few moments will often expand, deepen, and inspire the quality of consciousness that we and the teams we work with bring to a day's effort.

▼▼ In a real sense all life is inter-related. All persons are caught in an inescapable network of mutuality, tied in a single garment of destiny.

Whatever affects one directly affects all indirectly. I can never be what I ought to be until you are what you ought to be, and you can never be what you ought to be until I am what I ought to be. This is the inter-related structure of reality.

Martin Luther King, Jr.

THE "GOD CONVERSATION"

▼▼ Spirit... is the point of human transcendence; it is the point where the human is open to the Divine, that is, to the infinite and the eternal. It is also the point where human beings communicate. At that point of the Spirit we are all open to one another.

Father Bede Griffiths

Walking into the crowded meeting room at Bretton Woods conference center in Vermont, the first words we heard were, "Invoked or not, God is present." Surprised and delighted by the implications of this statement at a business conference, we pulled up a seat and joined the circle. Looking around, we found ourselves amid more than two hundred of our colleagues in rapt attention as M.I.T. learning organization specialist Peter Senge, Shell Oil executive Joe Jaworski, and journalist Betty Sue Flowers engaged in a passionate and heartfelt fishbowl dialogue. The dialogue began with the opening question, "What sort of interesting conversations are you having with leaders in business these days?" The first reply, "How about the 'God Conversation'? It's sure a hot topic these days."

As Peter put it, "All this systems stuff has no meaning without under-standing that we're part of something larger than ourselves. If our work has an impact, it will bring us back into the natural order of things." Knowing that we are all part of the web of life, a sacred reality, gives our lives and our work a sense of roots and meaning. Any description of reality, be it modern or ancient, religious, mythological, or scientific can only offer us a story, par-tial and incomplete, about reality. The inquiry in business about building community, stewardship, core values, belonging, and spirit is about "real time, real stuff" that has profound implications for people organizations serious about business success, learning, sustainability, competitive advantage, and retention of high caliber people in critical times.

Speaking to the importance of disciplines of meditation, Peter recently said, "Increasingly, we're directly incorporating into our work different practices that have been around for a long time, such as various types of meditation. It started with the work on dialogue. We found that dialogue often involved silence, and so maybe we needed to actually cultivate the capacity to sit in silence. And guess what? That started to look a lot like traditional forms of meditation or contemplation. So we've become more and more out front about this, although it's always been there. Though we had been doing the work described in *The Fifth Discipline* for ten or fifteen years before the book was published, we hadn't used the word *discipline*. It was only in the writing of the book that it finally hit me that what we were talking about was discipline, in the very same spirit in which the word has been used in the creative arts or in spiritual traditions for thousands of years. People might have a potential or a talent, but they can't cultivate it without discipline."

3 CREATIVE INTELLIGENCE: THE DYNAMIC SYNERGY OF ACTIVE AND QUIET MIND SKILLS ▼ ▼ ▼

Physicists explore levels of matter; mystics explore levels of mind. What they have in common is that both levels lie beyond ordinary sense perception.

Fritjof Capra

Insights and inspirations emerge into our minds first as subtle, formless impressions, gossamer and transparent—so elusive that they are easily ignored. If our "quiet mind skills" are keen enough, however, even the subtlest emerging insights will be noticed and drawn into awareness. Once these impressions are brought onto the "screen" of conscious awareness, our "active mind skills" come into play, shaping and developing these spontaneous mental impressions into more clearly defined thoughts, images, and intentions that can be communicated to others and can guide our action and work in the world. One of the most skillful ways we have found to introduce meditation into the world of work is as a discipline that provides powerful tools for developing creative intelligence through this dynamic synergy of the active-creative-imaginative mind and the quiet-receptive-intuitive mind.

Active mind skills are best understood as the tools of our intellect and reasoning. They include intention or will, thinking and reasoning, and our faculties of creative imagination. These skills each play a role in creatively shaping or transforming information through the power of intention. They also give form and meaning to the flow of information and the chaos of our experience by creating order through the power of thought and imagination.

The active mind skills are vital to organizing and expressing our inner knowing, insights, feelings, and intentions, and for translating our thoughts and visions into language and action. Active mind skills help us make sense both of internal mental experience and of the perceived experience from our outer world, and to communicate our understanding to others.

The quiet mind skills represent a domain of powerful mental functions that are complementary to and essential for the effective use of the active mind skills. Quiet mind skills are primarily attentive or receptive mental functions that gather information through the faculty of mindful attention, sensing, and feeling. These involve the qualities of presence, receptivity, or "being" in contrast to the generative, or "doing" nature of the active mind skills.

By way of analogy, the active mind skills can be compared to the forms and patterns of clouds or matter that we can see or touch, and the dynamic forces of wind, water, or electromagnetism that move, organize, and shape them. In contrast, the subtler mental functions and brain states associated with the quiet mind are more "transparent," like the sheer presence of the sky—vast in scope, clear, and open. For this reason they are rarely recognized, and seldom fully developed.

Although little if any attention is usually given to developing quiet mind skills in our formal education process or even professional training, the level of development and skill in this domain determines the coherence and power of all of our other mental functions. Critically important to accessing and expressing a deeper quality of wisdom and presence in our lives, the depth of our quiet mind skills determines our capacity for spaciously holding the intensity and complexity of our lives. Key to integrating both intellect and intuition, these quiet mind skills provide access to the subtle revelations of intuitive insight so crucial for breakthroughs in creativity and innovation.

Consciously or unconsciously, all the great scientists and sages of the world have tapped the quiet-receptive-intuitive mind to discover the universal organizing principles that have inspired and guided the development of humanity throughout the ages. By allowing us to focus our attention more deeply, quiet mind skills enable us to discover a more fundamental wisdom that reveals insight into the nature of our innermost being and the world in which we live. In this way, the quiet mind awakens our sensitivity to life-giving forces that are expressed as universal values, such as wisdom, kindness, compassion, and wonder.

Though few people have received any disciplined or rigorous formal training in either the active or quiet mind skills, all of us, to some degree, rely on these complementary faculties each day to make sense of our experience and to organize our thinking and working. In fact, the quality of our work, communication, thinking, creativity, and health are intimately related to how fully we have developed the dynamic synergy of these two kinds of mental capabilities.

Begin to experiment with bringing more conscious awareness and skill to the balanced interplay of these mind states. As you talk, also deeply listen. Observe and sense how images and associations actively cascade through the space of the quiet receptive mind like clouds forming and disappearing when warm moist winds pass over a ridge in the high mountains. Notice how the active foreground display of your abstract thoughts or imaginings emerges and shapes itself against the backdrop of quiet mindful awareness. Within this deep stillness of the mind, experience how images arise, develop, and dissolve back into the open clear field of primordial awareness.

The different styles of meditation practice presented throughout this book have all been designed to provide you with the kind of "mental fitness" training that will help you cultivate your capacity to integrate these two vital dimensions of creative intelligence into your daily life and work.

4 PROFOUNDLY INSPIRED WORK:
VISIONARY RESEARCH▼ ▼ ▼

There is no inspiration
without aspiration.
      Rabindranath Tagore

For us, one of the most inspiring examples of revealing the sacred dimensions of life through work was our experience coaching the team of a pioneering two-year "visionary research" project that we helped support at the Weyerhaeuser company. Understanding that research methods could be dramatically accelerated by tapping intuition and developing creative intelligence, Jon Dunnington, the program leader, invited us to coach his team in the personal and team skills necessary to succeed in "visionary research." The intent of this project was to discover and demonstrate the power and potential of new ways of thinking and knowing that could help research and development teams achieve a higher level of performance and make breakthroughs that would help build a better world. We took to heart Einstein's statement that, "The world we have made as a result of the level of the thinking we have done thus far creates problems that we cannot solve at the same level at which we have created them... We shall require a substantially new manner of thinking if humankind is to survive."

The methods we used were essentially methods for quieting, focusing, and opening the mind, seeding it with a clear question—a yearning, a prayer—and then being present to listen deeply and intuitively for the inspirations that would arise. Over time the group developed protocols blending methods of relaxation, concentration, and meditation plus a rather prayerful yearning to bring forth innovations that would truly be good for the world.

For two years, the members of our team met every other week to search for breakthrough ideas to the myriad special research projects going on within various departments. As the members of our research team became more adept at the inner practices, they learned to, individually and collectively, tap their wellsprings of intuitive intelligence and inspiration. The results were astonishing in a number of ways, personally and institutionally. We learned that the questions we held in our minds would organize our attention, and that the quality and scope of our individual and shared intention determined the bandwidth of possibilities and applications that were revealed through our inquiry. People on the team were inspired and excited by the consistency of the team's results and the implications for reliably accessing breakthroughs in creativity and innovation at many settings around the globe.

"Our questions were at times like heartfelt prayers," one person said. "In the silence of our deep listening together, it was as though each of us had learned to push the pause button on the stories we keep telling ourselves about who we are. In this state of deep shared listening, we'd converge like islands meeting at their common roots deep under the surface of the sea, merging within a larger field of Presence in which we are both one and many."

Here's one example of our visionary research process on this project. The session leader working on an aquaculture project discussed his quandary over the disappointing rate of spawning salmon in rehabilitated streams that had been stocked. No one knew why so few salmon were returning.

In search of clues, he invited us to join him on an imaginary journey through the life cycle of a salmon. He painted a vivid picture of our life in the hatchery, the day we were loaded into a truck and set loose in the river. Then as we approached the mouth of the river and encountered salt water for the first time, he set our imagination and intuition loose to explore the many forces that might shape our lives as salmon and determine if we would return to spawn or not.

Surfacing from this long, deep dive, we took time to jot or doodle our impressions and then to discuss insights that had come to mind. Some of us described the trauma of being loaded and unloaded into the truck that took us from the hatchery to the river. Others had valuable insights regarding moving from fresh water into the salt water or the open ocean. Still others offered possible clues about conditions at sea that might affect our life cycle and spawning rates. Together these many pieces formed a picture that offered an inspiring number of valuable and unexpected insights for where to look to improve the conditions necessary for increasing the successful release and return of the salmon. Similar intuitive approaches consistently proved fruitful on many other projects related to forest products, land management, and resource issues over the years that we worked together.

Working in this way, each person's insights offered a clue or elicited an insight from others. Our inquiry would build naturally upon itself like atoms coalescing into a complex thought molecule, ideas cascading from question to intuition to explanation to application in an effortless, superconductive way.

The answers to our questions were often surprising and unexpected. Brother David Steindl-Rast has said, "Another name for God is surprise!" At times this notion rang so true that we were stunned into a deeply reverent shared silence. Often we talked about what it would be like to harness the power unleashed by the joy and wonder in this work, and focus these individual and collective skills toward addressing some of the really big challenges facing humanity. At times we sensed that our research work—this remarkable experiment in deep, shared intuitive inquiry—was creating a story that would offer inspiration, courage, and guidance for other research and development teams for decades to come.

Though the challenges were great, the ocean of inspiration seemed intent on splashing itself into our minds as a deeply intuitive knowing that would weave its way into our thinking and dreaming, providing business solutions that mere analysis or laboratory research could never have yielded. This research gave rise to inspiring innovations, many of which carried significant bottom-line benefits for the business and enhanced the quality of life for people and for the environment.

5 GLIMPSING THE SACRED
IN DAILY WORK-LIFE▼ ▼ ▼

Ethics is how we behave when we decide we belong together.
Brother David Steindl-Rast

A colleague at the Harvard Business School commented that they are seeing an increasingly compelling yearning among people to integrate the spiritual dimensions of their lives into their work in the world. People are beginning to realize that if they are going to spend a large part of their lives in the office and on the job, they want their time to be rewarding spiritually as well as materially. We have found that one way to honor this yearning and to understand how Spirit manifests in the workplace is to invite a dialogue with people you work with to inquire, "When, or how, do we glimpse Spirit at work?" Responses we have heard include:

▼ In moments of caring, kindness, and compassion.
▼ In moments of deep listening or in shared silence.
▼ In moments of clarity, when we glimpse our place in the "big picture."
▼ In moments of wonder, when synchronicities converge to confirm our intuition with a "yes!"
▼ In moments of collaboration, when we join forces to create a better world.
▼ In mindful moments, when we are wholeheartedly present.
▼ In moments of deep recognition of each other and of ourselves.
▼ In moments of dialogue, when synergy reveals a glimpse of truth larger than one person can hold.

▼ In moments of forgiveness, when we let go of the past and focus on creating our future.

▼ In moments of commitment, when our love and action blend into one.

▼▼ People are hungry for ways in which to practice spirituality in the workplace without offending their coworkers or causing acrimony. They believe strongly that unless organizations learn to how to harness the "whole person" and the immense spiritual energy that is at the core of everyone, they will not be able to produce world-class products and services.

Sloan Management Review

6 DATA TO INSPIRE FAITH ▼ ▼ ▼

And I have felt a presence that disturbs me
with the joy of elevated thoughts;
a sense sublime of something far more deeply interfused,
whose dwelling is the light of setting suns,
and the round ocean and the living air,
and the blue sky, and in the mind of man;
A motion and a spirit, that impels
All thinking things, all objects of thought,
And rolls through all things.

William Wordsworth

In our work with people from around the globe we are continually heartened to see a growing understanding that both individuals and organizations would be wise to develop their resilience and capacity to meet the challenges and opportunities of these turbulent times. With increasing frequency we find people interested in learning more about improving their health, enhancing their performance, increasing ethical impeccability, deepening their emotional intelligence, cultivating mindfulness, learning more personal mastery skills, bringing a deeper wisdom to work, and integrating spiritual values, principles, and practices more fully into their lives. A growing interest in spirituality as it relates to values, health, business, and the whole of life is evident in recent polls and articles in *Industry Week, Business Week, Journal of the American Medical Association, Fortune, Newsweek, New Leaders,* the *New York Times,* and *Leaders* magazines and the recent *International Workplace*

Values Survey, which involved 1,200 people in eighteen countries around the world.

Each year it seems that there are more major conferences for leaders in business that have a specific focus on integrating more soul or spirit into business. Confirming these trends, the Institute for the Future located in Northern California launched a project to document the increasingly important role of spirituality in business. This is an exciting time when more and more people are recognizing that if we are to live sustainably on this planet we must attend more carefully to the health and wholeness of ourselves and our world.

Among the organizations that are leading the way in this important integral work are the Society for Organizational Learning, the Institute of Noetic Sciences, the World Business Academy, the Center for Mindfulness & Medicine at the University of Massachusetts Medical School, the Sante Fe Institute, California Institute of Integral Studies, Princeton Engineering Anomalies Research Project at Princeton's School of Engineering, Case Western Reserve University Medical School's Institute for Research on Unlimited Love, the International Society for the Study of Subtle Energies and Energy Medicine, Contemplative Mind in Society, and the Fetzer Foundation. We invite you to seek these institutions out online and to follow links from their websites that will carry you into a vast network of inspiring resources and insights.

To get a feeling for the findings of the recent polls on how people find balance through spirituality, imagine yourself out on the town, at work, or at a community meeting. See yourself surrounded by all of your coworkers, partners, customers, and suppliers, or by all your neighbors. Then, as you look around at all these people, keep in mind that the polls say that two out of three of these people have a deep yearning for spiritual growth. Fifty-five percent of us have experienced a "personal transformation" in recent years. Eighty percent of us believe in God, and three out of four of us believe that unexplainable miracles are a reality in our lives. Ninety percent of us reach out to the sacred through prayer or meditation, and 57 percent of us pray daily. The 2001 Spirituality & Health National Poll indicated that 84 percent of Americans view God as being "everywhere and in everything" rather than "someone somewhere," reminding us that every person and every situation of our life-work can be approached in a sacred manner.

Even if we don't talk about it, or have the right words to describe it, there have been instants in most of our lives when, for a timeless moment, the fabric of the story we tell ourselves dissolved to reveal that, in truth, we are both particle *and* wave, wave *and* ocean. Fully a third of us—your friends, family, and coworkers—have had a profound or life-altering religious or mystical experience. In reality, the mystery or spirit is as close to us as water is to waves. As Saul demonstrated on the road to Damascus, and as countless others have experienced playing sports, giving birth, or driving down the road on the way to work, we are utterly unable to protect ourselves from spontaneous moments of grace.

For millennia, the world's great wisdom traditions have empirically tested and refined myriad effective inner technologies that consistently increase the incidence of close encounters with the sacred—if you practice them. Just as some people have yet to log on to the Internet or surf the Web, the priorities of our lives or the limited scope of our inquiry have left some of us still quite unaware of the wealth of resources within and around us for discovering, living, and working in a more soulful, spirited, and multidimensional way.

If you need more incentive for establishing a meditation practice, then keep in mind that the growing body of research on health and high-level human performance shows that people who have a spiritual orientation and have cultivated a greater sense of their wholeness are more change and stress resilient, and more creative and productive. There is considerable evidence suggesting that having a spiritual orientation toward life offers benefits both for individuals and for businesses.

After five years of study in many leading corporations, Stanford University's pioneering Corporate Health Program project, funded by the Rockefeller Foundation, concluded that a spiritual orientation toward life increases our change resilience and is one of five characteristics that are the basis for "optimal health." The World Workplace Values Survey tells us that interest in spiritual development ranks ahead of physical development in its importance to people in business, leading us to rethink the facilities and perks that may best reward our staffs. Clinical studies indicate that people who are sick are 75 percent more likely to become better if they have a spiritual view of life. In alcohol treatment, a "spiritual change" in a person is associated with a 93 percent lasting sobriety rate.

If you take these thoughts to heart you may discover that you are more than the story you've been telling yourself. Much more. Your thoughts are the creative display of your deeper reality. Don't mistake the story for the truth. The reality of your soulfulness is at work or play in every moment; it is here as the silence amid sounds and as the stillness within ceaseless motion; as the clarity within confusion, and the knowingness at the heart of your unknowing. Each day the tides of hope and fear, beauty and pain, break open our minds. The breakthroughs and breakdowns of life and work break open our hearts and help us to wake up, to remember who we really are.

For some of us, scientific research inspires our faith that spirit is alive in our daily lives, even if we seldom discuss it. These findings are useful to seed conversations with your family, friends, and coworkers about the beliefs and core values that are truly at the heart of our lives. As more and more people are seeking for balance in their lives, it seems that no relationship, family, business, or organization can afford to disregard or deplete the vitality, creativity, productivity, passion, and creative spirit of its people. These rare and precious human resources of the creative human spirit are clearly necessary for sustained success in every arena of our personal, professional, and shared lives.

RESOURCES

▼▼ When you practice these
precious teachings, slowly the clouds of
sorrow melt away. And the sun
of wisdom and true joy will be shining
in the clear sky of your mind.
Kalu Rinpoche

SUGGESTED FURTHER READINGS AND RESOURCES

RELAXATION

Borysenko, Joan. *Inner Peace for Busy People*. Carlsbad, CA: Hay House, 2001.

Benson, Herbert. *The Relaxation Response*. New York: Avon, 1976.

———. *Beyond the Relaxation Response*. New York: Berkley, 1984.

Davis, Martha, et al. *The Relaxation and Stress Reduction Workbook*. Oakland, CA: New Harbinger Publications, 2000.

George, Mike. *Learn to Relax*. San Francisco: Chronicle Books, 1998.

Harvey, John R. *Total Relaxation*. New York: Kodansha International, 1998.

Levey, Joel. *The Fine Art of Relaxation: Self-Guided CD*. Seattle: EarthView, 2000.

Levey, Joel and Michelle. *A Moment to Relax*. San Francisco: Cronicle Books, 2003.

Tarthang Tulku. *Kum Nye Relaxation*. Berkeley: Dharma, 1978.

CONCENTRATION

Feurstein, Georg. *The Yoga-Sutra of Patanjali*. Rochester, VT: Inner Traditions, 1990.

Feurstein, Georg and Ken Wilber. *The Yoga Tradition: History, Religion, Philosophy and Practice*. Prescott, AZ: Hohm Press, 2001.

Gunaratana, Henepola. *The Path of Serenity and Insight*, Delhi: Motilal Banarsidass, 1985.

Iyengar, B. K. S. *Light on Pranayama: The Yogic Art of Breathing*. New York: Crossroad/Herder & Herder, 1995.

Lati Rinbochay; Denma Lochö Rinbochay; Zahler, Leah; and Hopkins, Jeffrey. *Meditative States in Tibetan Buddhism*. London: Wisdom, 1983.

Levey, Joel and Michelle. *The Focused Mindstate: Maximizing Your Potential through the Power of Concentration*. Seven-tape album with workbook. Chicago: Nightingale-Conant, 1993.

Nhat Hanh, Thich. *The Long Road Turns to Joy: A Guide to Walking Meditation*. Berkeley: Parallax Press, 1996.

Taimni, I. K. *The Science of Yoga.* Wheaton: Theosophical Publishing House, A Quest Book, 1961.

Vivekananda, Swami. *Raja Yoga.* New York: Ramakrishna-Vivekananda Center, 1973.

Buddhaghosa. *The Path of Purification*, Trans. Bhikkhu Nanamoli. Kandy, Sri Lanka: Buddhist Publication Society, 1979.

MEDITATION

Barks, Coleman, and Michael Gree. *The Illuminated Rumi.* New York: Doubleday, 1997.

Berzin, Alexander. *Developing Balanced Sensitivity.* Ithaca: Snow Lion, 1998.

Blofeld, John. *The Zen Teachings of Huang Po.* New York: Grove, 1959.

Boorstein, Sylvia. *Don't Just Do Something, Sit There: A Mindfulness Retreat.* San Francisco: Harper, 1996.

Borysenko, Joan. *Fire in the Soul: A New Psychology of Spiritual Optimism.* New York: Warner Books, 1993.

———. *Meditations for Overcoming Depression.* Carson, CA: Hay House Audio, 1995.

Byrom, Thomas, trans. *The Dhammapada: The Sayings of the Buddha.* New York: Vintage, 1976.

Chödron, Pema. *When Things Fall Apart.* Boston: Shambhala, 1997.

———. *The Places That Scare You: A Guide to Fearlessness in Difficult Times.* Boston: Shambhala, 2001.

———. *Start Where You Are: A Guide to Compassionate Living.* Boston: Shambhala, 1994.

Chödron, Thubten. *Working with Anger.* Ithaca: Snow Lion, 2001.

Dalai Lama. *Ethics for a New Millennium.* New York: Putnam, 1999.

———. *Dzogchen: The Heart Essence of the Great Perfection.* Ithaca: Snow Lion, 2000.

Dalai Lama; Keily, Robert; and Freeman, Dom Laurence. *The Good Heart: A Buddhist Perspective on the Teachings of Jesus.* Boston: Wisdom Publications, 1998.

Das, Surya. *Awakening the Buddha Within.* New York: Broadway Books, 1997.

Dass, Ram. *Grist for the Mill.* Santa Cruz: Unity, 1977.

———. *Journey of Awakening.* New York: Bantam, 1978.

de Mello, Anthony. *Sadhana: A Way to God, Christian Exercises in Eastern Form.* New York: Doubleday, 1984.

———. *Awareness.* Image Books, 1990.

———. *The Heart of the Enlightened: A Book of Story Meditations.* Image Books, 1991.

————. *The Way to Love.* Image Books, 1995.

————. *Praying Body and Soul: Principles, Practices, Stories.* New York: Crossroads, 1997.

Dilgo Khyentse Rinpoche. *Enlightened Courage.* Ithaca: Snow Lion, 1994.

Dossey, Larry. *Healing Words: The Power of Prayer and the Practice of Medicine.* New York: HarperCollins, 1993.

————. *Prayer Is Good Medicine.* New York: HarperCollins, 1996.

Eppsteiner, Fred; and Dennis Maloney, eds. *The Path of Compassion: Contemporary Writings on Engaged Buddhism.* Berkeley: Parallax, 1988.

Feurstein, Georg and Ken Wilber. *The Yoga Tradition: History, Religion, Philosophy and Practice.* Prescott, AZ: Holm Press, 2001.

Fox, Mathew. *A Spirituality Named Compassion.* San Francisco: Harper & Row, 1992.

Fryba, Mirko. *The Art of Happiness: Teachings of Buddhist Psychology.* Boston: Shambhala, 1989.

Glassman, Bernie. *Bearing Witness: A Zen Master's Lessons in Making Peace.* New York: Bell Tower, 1998.

Glassman, Bernard and Rick Fields. *Instructions to the Cook: A Zen Master's Lessons in Living a Life That Matters.* New York: Random House, 1997.

Goldstein, Joseph. *Insight Meditation: The Practice of Freedom.* Boston: Shambhala, 1993.

Govinda, Lama Anagarika. *Creative Meditation and Multidimensional Consciousness.* Wheaton: Theosophical Publishing House, 1976.

Griffiths, Bede. *A New Vision of Reality: Western Science, Eastern Mysticism, and Christian Faith.* Springfield, IL: Templegate, 1990.

Handelsman, Judith. *Growing Myself: A Spiritual Journey Through Gardening.* New York: Dutton, 1996.

Helminski, Kabir Edmund. *Living Presence: A Sufi Way to Mindfulness and the Essential Self.* Los Angeles: J. P. Tarcher, 1992.

————. *The Knowing Heart: A Sufi Path of Transformation.* Boston: Shambhala, 2000.

Hixon, Lex. *Sufi Meditation.* Westport, CT: Pir Publications, 1997.

Kabat-Zinn, Jon. *Wherever You Go, There You Are: Mindfulness Meditation in Everyday Life.* New York: Hyperion, 1994.

Kabat-Zinn, Jon and Myla. *Everyday Blessings: The Inner Work of Mindful Parenting.* New York: Hyperion, 1997.

Kalu Rinpoche. *The Dharma That Illuminates All Beings Impartially Like the Light of the Sun and the Moon.* Albany: SUNY, 1986.

Kaplan, Aryeh. *Jewish Meditation: A Practical Guide.* New York: Schocken, 1985.

Keating, Thomas. *Open Mind, Open Heart: The Contemplative Dimension of the Gospel.* New York: HarperCollins, 1994.

Kelly, Jack and Marcia. *Sanctuaries: The West Coast and Southwest Guide to Lodgings in Monasteries, Abbeys, and Retreats of the United States.* New York: Bell Tower, 1996.

Khalsa, Dharma Singh and Cameron Stauth. *Meditation As Medicine.* New York: Pocket Books, 2001.

Kornfield, Jack. *A Path with Heart: A Guide through the Perils and Promises of Spiritual Life.* New York: Bantam, 1993.

Krishnamurti, J. *Meditations.* Boston: Shambhala, 1979.

Labowitz, Rabbi Shoni. *Miraculous Living.* New York: Simon and Schuster, 1996.

Lao Tzu. *Tao Te Ching.* Trans. Gia-fu Feng and Jane English. New York: Vintage, 1974.

Levey, Joel and Michelle. *Simple Meditation & Relaxation.* Berkeley: Conari Press, 1999.

———. *Wisdom at Work: A Treasure of Tools for Cultivating Clarity, Kindness, and Resilience.* Berkeley: Conari Press, 1999.

———. *Living in Balance: A Dynamic Approach for Creating Harmony and Wholeness in a Chaotic World.* Berkeley: Conari Press, 1998.

Levine, Stephen. *A Gradual Awakening.* New York: Anchor-Doubleday, 1989.

———. *Who Dies? An Investigation of Conscious Living and Conscious Dying.* New York: Anchor-Doubleday, 1989.

———. *Turning toward the Mystery: A Seeker's Journey.* New York: Harper Collins, 2002.

Levine, Stephen and Ondrea. *Embracing the Beloved: Relationship As a Path of Awakening.* New York: Doubleday, 1995.

Macy, Joanna and Molly Young Brown. *Coming Back to Life: Practices to Reconnect Our Lives, Our World.* Gabriola Is., Canada: New Society Publishers, 1998.

McDonald, Kathleen. *How to Meditate.* Boston: Wisdom, 1989.

McLeod, Ken. *Wake Up To Your Life.* San Francisco: Harper San Francisco, 2001.

Merton, Thomas. *Contemplation in a World of Action.* New York: Doubleday, 1973.

———. *New Seeds of Contemplation.* New York: New Directions, 1976.

Mitchell, Stephen, ed. *The Enlightened Heart: An Anthology of Sacred Poetry.* New York: Harper & Row, 1989.

Moore, Thomas. *Care of the Soul: A Guide for Cultivating Depth and Sacredness in Everyday Life.* New York: HarperCollins, 1992.

Muller, Wayne. *Sabbath.* New York: Bantam, 1999.

Namgyal, Takpo Tashi. *Mahamudra: The Quintessence of Mind and Meditation.* Trans. Lobsang Lhalungpa. Boston: Shambhala, 1986.

Nhat Hanh, Thich. *Miracle of Mindfulness*. Boston: Beacon, 1984.

———. *Being Peace*. Berkeley: Parallax, 1987.

———. *The Heart of Understanding*. Berkeley: Parallax, 1988.

———. *Peace Is Every Step*. New York: Bantam Books, 1991.

———. *For a Future to Be Possible*. Berkeley: Parallax, 1993.

Norbu, Namkhai. *The Crystal and the Way of Light: Sutra, Tantra, and Dzogchen*. London: Routledge & Kegan Paul, 1986.

———. *The Supreme Source*. Ithaca: Snow Lion, 1999.

Reps, Paul. *Zen Flesh, Zen Bones*. Boston: Shambhala, 1994.

Rozman, Deborah. *Meditating with Children*. Boulder Creek: University of the Trees, 1977.

Salzberg, Sharon. *Voices of Insight*. Boston: Shambhala, 1991.

———. *Lovingkindness: The Revolutionary Art of Happiness*. Boston: Shambhala, 1997.

———. *A Heart As Wide As the World*. Boston: Shambhala, 1997.

———. *Faith*. Boston:Shambhala, 2002.

Schachter-Shalomi, Zalman. *The First Step: A Guide for the New Jewish Spirit*. New York: Bantam, 1983.

Sogyal Rinpoche. *The Tibetan Book of Living and Dying*. San Francisco: Harper, 1992.

Steindl-Rast, Brother David. *Gratefulness: The Heart of Prayer*. New York: Paulist Press, 1984.

Sudo, Philip Sud. *Zen Computer: Mindfulness and the Machine.*. New York: Simon & Schuster, 2000.

Suzuki, Shunryu. *Zen Mind, Beginner's Mind*. New York: Weatherhill, 1986.

Tart, Charles. *Living the Mindful Life: A Handbook for Living in the Present Moment*. Boston: Shambhala, 1994.

Tarthang Tulku. *Space Time and Knowledge*. Berkeley: Dharma, 1977.

———. *Gesture of Balance*. Berkeley: Dharma, 1977.

———. *Knowledge of Freedom*. Berkeley: Dharma, 1984.

———. *Love of Knowledge*. Berkeley: Dharma, 1987.

———. *Sacred Dimensions of Time and Space*. Berkeley: Dharma, 1998.

Thondup Tulku and Daniel Goleman. *The Healing Power of the Mind: Simple Exercises for Health, Well-being, and Enlightenment*. Boston: Shambhala, 1998.

Thurman, Robert. *Inner Revolution*. New York: Riverhead, 1998.

Tolle, Eckhart. *The Power of Now*. Novato, CA: New World Library, 1999.

Trungpa, Chogyam. *Shambhala: The Sacred Path of the Warrior.* Boston: Shambhala, 1984.

Ueshiba, Morihei. *The Art of Peace.* Trans. John Stevens. Boston: Shambhala, 1992.

Walker, Brian. *Hua Hu Ching: The Unknown Teachings of Lao Tsu.* San Francisco: Harper San Francisco, 1992.

Yeshe, Thubten. *Introduction to Tantra.* Boston: Wisdom, 1989.

Ywahoo, Dhyani. *Voices of Our Ancestors: Cherokee Teachings from the Wisdom Fire.* Boston: Shambhala, 1987.

BIOGRAPHIES

Allione, Tsultrim. *Women of Wisdom.* London: Arkana, 1986.

Dalai Lama. *Freedom in Exile: The Autobiography of the Dalai Lama.* New York: Harper-Collins, 1990.

Du Boulay, Shirley. *Beyond the Darkness: A Biography of Bede Griffiths.* New York: Doubleday, 2002.

Govinda, Lama Anagarika. *The Way of the White Clouds.* Boston: Shambhala, 1970.

Gyatso, Janet. *Apparitions of the Self: The Secret Autobiographies of a Tibetan Visionary.* Princeton: Princeton University Press, 1998.

Kalu Rinpoche. *The Chariot for Travelling the Path to Freedom: The Life Story of Kalu Rinpoche.* Trans. Kenneth McLeod. San Francisco: Kagyu Dharma, 1985.

Lhalungpa, Lobsang. *The Life of Milarepa.* Boston: Shambhala, 1984.

Macy, Joanna. *Widening Circles.* Gabriola Is., B.C.: New Society Publishers, 2000.

Mackenzie, Vicki. *The Boy Lama.* San Francisco: Harper & Row, 1988.

Merrell-Wolff, Franklin. *Pathways through Space.* New York: Julian, 1973.

Nhat Hanh, Thich. *Old Path, White Clouds.* Berkeley: Parallax Press, 1991.

Roach, Michael. *The Diamond Cutter: The Buddha on Strategies for Managing Your Business and Your Life.* New York: Doubleday, 2000.

Roberts, Bernadette. *The Experience of No-Self.* Boston: Shambhala, 1984.

——. *The Path to No-Self: Life at the Center.* Boston: Shambhala, 1985.

Tarthang Tulku. *Mother of Knowledge.* Berkeley: Dharma, 1983.

Thurman, Robert and Tad Wise. *Circling the Sacred Mountain.* New York: Bantam, 1999.

Tweedie, Irina. *Daughter of Fire: A Diary of a Spiritual Training with a Sufi Master.* Inverness, CA: Golden Sufi Center, 1995.

Ullman, Robert and Judyth Riechenberg Ullman. *Mystics, Masters, Saints, & Sages.* Berkeley: Conari Press, 2000.

Yogananda, Paramahansa. *Autobiography of a Yogi*. Los Angeles: Self Realization Fellowship Pub, 1985.

EXTRAORDINARY PERFORMANCE

Grey, Alex. *Sacred Mirrors: The Visionary Art of Alex Grey*. Rochester, VT: Inner Traditions, 1990.

———. *Transfigurations*. Rochester, VT: Inner Traditions, 2001.

Csikszentmihalyi, Mihaly. *Flow: The Psychology of Optimal Experience*. New York: Harper & Row, 1990.

———. *Creativity: Flow and the Psychology of Discovery and Invention*. New York: HarperCollins, 1996.

Dass, Ram and Paul Gorman. *How Can I Help? Stories and Reflections on Service*. New York: Alfred A. Knopf, 1990.

Garfield, Charles. *Peak Performance New Heroes of American Business*. New York: Avon, 1991.

Garfield, Charles and Hal Bennett. *Peak Performance: Mental Training Techniques of the World's Greatest Athletes*. Los Angeles: Warner, 1989.

Harman, Willis and Howard Rheingold. *Higher Creativity: Liberating the Unconscious for Breakthrough Insights*. Los Angeles: Tarcher, 1984.

Heckler, Richard Strozzi. *Aikido and the New Warrior*. Berkeley: North Atlantic, 1985.

Ingram, Catherine. *In the Footsteps of Gandhi: Conversations with Spiritual Social Activists*. Berkeley: Parallax, 1989.

Murphy, Michael. *The Future of the Body: Explorations into the Further Evolution of Human Nature*. Los Angeles: Tarcher, 1992.

Murphy, Michael and Rhea White. *In the Zone: Transcendent Experience in Sports*. New York: Penguin, 1995.

Treece, Patricia. *The Sanctified Body*. New York: Doubleday, 1987.

Weber, Renee. *Dialogues with Scientists and Sages: The Search for Unity*. London: Arkana, 1990.

CONSCIOUSNESS RESEARCH AND CREATIVITY

Austin, James. *Zen & the Brain*. Cambridge: MIT Press, 1999.

Dalai Lama. *Consciousness at the Crossroads: Conversations with the Dalai Lama on Brainscience and Buddhism*.Edited by Zara Houshmand, et al. Ithaca: Snow Lion, 1999.

Dalai Lama; Benson, Herbert; Thurman, Robert; and Goleman, Daniel. *Mind Science: An East-West Dialogue*. Boston: Shambhala, 1991.

Davidson, Richard and Anne Harrington, eds. *Visions of Compassion: Western Scientists and Tibetan Buddhists Examine Human Nature*. New York: Oxford Press, 2001.

Dossey, Larry. *Recovering the Soul: A Scientific and Spiritual Search*. New York: Bantam, 1989.

―――. *Healing beyond the Body: Medicine and the Infinite Reach of the Mind*. Boston: Shambhala, 2001.

Goleman, Daniel. *Emotional Intelligence*. New York: Bantam, 1997.

――― *Healing Emotions*. Boston: Shambhala, 1997.

Jahn, Robert G. and Brenda J. Dunne. *Margins of Reality: The Role of Consciousness in the Physical World*. San Diego: Harvest Books, 1987.

Murphy, Michael and Steven Donovan. *The Physical and Psychological Effects of Meditation*. Sausalito, CA: Institute of Noetic Science, 1990.

Newberg, Andrew and Eugene d'Aquili. *Why God Won't Go Away: Brain Science and the Biology of Belief*. New York: Ballantine, 2001.

Radin, Dean. *The Conscious Universe: The Scientific Truth of Psychic Phenomena*. San Francisico: Harper, 1997.

Tiller, William A. *Science and Human Transformation*. Walnut Creek, CA: Pavior, 1997.

Wilber, Ken; Brown, Daniel; and Engler, Jack. *Transformations of Consciousness: Conventional and Contemplative Developmental Approaches*. Boston: Shambhala, 1986.

WEBSITES OF INTEREST

We invite you to explore the following websites in order to deepen your insight regarding the profoundly practical applications and integration of contemplative practices and associated advances in mindsciences into the many domains of our modern lives.

- Archives of Scientists' Transcendent Experiences: www.issc-taste.org

- Center for Contemplative Mind in Society: www.contemplativemind.org

- Christianity & Science: http://search.netscape.com/Science/Science_in_Society/Science_and_Religion/Christianity_and_Science

- Dharma Seed Archival Center. Excellent source of taped lectures and meditation teachings. Streaming audio on-line: www.Dhamastream.org

- Inquiring Mind. Excellent, contemporary newsletter on meditation and mindfulness retreats: www.inquiringmind.com

- Institute of Noetic Sciences. Excellent source of research and integration of contemplative principles and practices in science, medicine, business, and other domains of contemporary life: www.noetic.org

- International Society for the Study of Subtle Energy and Energy Medicine (ISSSEEM). Excellent source of research on healing arts and energy medicine: www.issseem.org

- Monastic Interreligious Dialogue: www.osb.org/mid/ and at www.monasticdialog.org/

- New Dimensions Radio. Excellent source of audiotape interviews with leaders in mindbody-spirit research and health: www.newdimensions.org

- Princeton Engineering Anomalies Research (PEAR) Scientific Study of Consciousness-Related Physical Phenomena. Engineering and Consciousness: www.princeton.edu/~pear/

- Science & Spirit research archives: www.science-spirit.org/resnews/resnews.cfm

- Sounds True Catalogue. Excellent source of audio recordings related to mindbody-spirit: www.soundstrue.com

- The Mind and Life Institute. Good source of research and insights: www.mindandlife.org

- University of Arizona Center for Consciousness Studies: Excellent source of latest current scientific research on consciousness: www.consciousness.arizona.edu

ACKNOWLEDGMENTS

The interest, enthusiasm, and devoted work of many fine people have brought this book into multiple editions and languages. Originally, this material emerged as a collection of training materials and handouts that we created while we were running clinical programs in various medical centers. Over the years this book has continued to evolve, expand, and be a source of guidance and inspiration for an ever widening circle of people around the globe.

Our thanks to the many people at Wisdom Publications who have contributed their vision, skill, dedication, and artistry to the evolution of this book in its various editions. In particular, we'd like to acknowledge Nick Ribush for his original inspiration and selection of *The Fine Arts of Relaxation, Concentration, and Meditation* as the first of Wisdom's East West Series, and also Pamela Cowan and Steve Miller for bringing this manuscript to Nick's attention.

On an inner level, the profound depth of wisdom, ethical impeccability, and compassionate activity of our many teachers have profoundly inspired, and in countless ways contributed to, this book. We give special thanks to His Holiness Tenzin Gyatso the Dalai Lama; Kyabje Zong Rinpoche; Venerable Kalu Rinpoche; Lama Thubten Yeshe; Venerable Gen Lamrimpa; Rina Sircar; Sogyal Rinpoche; and Chagdud Rinpoche for the inspiration of their living examples. Their methods of teaching and their careful guidance of our own practice of these inner arts have deeply touched our hearts and opened our minds to new dimensions of understanding.

Inspiration for this book has also come from the 16th Karmapa, Brother David Steindl-Rast, Rabbi Shlomo Carlbach, Lama Govinda, Geshe Ngawang Dhargye, Dezhung Rinpoche, Dagchen Rinpoche, Geshe Gyeltsen, Zasep Rinpoche, Soen Sa Nim, Dipama, Goenka, Taungpulu Sayadaw, Rabbi Zalman Shachter, Pir Vilayat Khan, Reshad Field, Thich Nhat Hanh, Dhyani Ywahoo, Sasaki Roshi, and many others with whom we have been fortunate to study.

Holding lineages of teachings that have been cherished and preserved for millennia, these teachers have conveyed a living transmission of ancient wisdom into modern times. In recent years, many of these remarkable teachers have died. If in some way this book contributes to the continued understanding and practice of the wisdom and altruistic concern that they so inspiringly embodied and taught, then our intentions will be fulfilled.

The friendship and skillful teaching styles of Ram Dass, Stephen Levine, Richard Barron, Jonathan Landaw, Joseph Goldstein, Jack Kornfield, Elmer Green, Bill Arnesen, Robert Hover, Angeles Arrien, Roger Walsh, Ruth Denison, John Kabat-Zinn, and Paul Reps have all inspired and energized aspects of our own teaching of these practices over the years.

Our heartfelt thanks also go to our many students, friends, and colleagues around the globe with whom we have shared and refined the presentation of these methods. We'd especially like to thank Alan Millar; Bill Veltrop; the HumanKind community; our colleagues from Menninger Foundation's Council Grove Conference; the International Center for Organization Design; the Institute for Noetic Sciences; our Hawaii *ohana*; and the many communities and organizations that we have worked and taught in for their encouragement and inspiration in developing this book.

We offer our deep appreciation and gratitude to Bryan Brewer at Earthview, Inc. (www.self-guided.com) for permission to adapt numerous tracks from Joel's compact disc *The Fine Art of Relaxation*; Taungpulu Sayadaw and Rina Sircar for permission to include the "Concentration while walking" exercise; and John Blofeld for the "Mother of compassion" meditation

Joel would also like to acknowledge his first teachers: his grandparents Hilda and Abe Levey, whose faith, humor, and kindness inspired him to value what he does; and his mother, Recia Millar, whose courage and determination to live was his first example of the power of faith, prayer, and devotion. Michelle acknowledges with heartfelt gratitude the steadfast support and teachings of her beloved parents, Ida and Benjamin Gold, from whom she has learned and received so much.

Through the wisdom and kindness of these and countless other people, the spirit of the inner technologies offered in this book has been woven deeply into the fabric of our lives. Now, through your own inquiry and practice of these methods, may the spirit within them come alive for you.

AUTHORS' BIOGRAPHY

JOEL LEVEY, PH.D., and MICHELLE LEVEY, M.A., have devoted their lives to intensive study and research of extra-ordinary human potential. Over the past thirty years they have been fortunate to study and practice with many of the greatest contemplative teachers of our times, and with many of the most respected researchers of human potential, mind sciences, and holistic medicine. Many of their mentors have encouraged them to teach what they have learned and they have translated their research and contemplative practice into active service with hundreds of organizations, businesses, medical centers, and communities around the globe.

Joel and Michelle are founders of InnerWork Technologies, Inc., a Seattle-based firm that specializes in developing and renewing organizational cultures in which life-work balance, high-performance teamwork, and resilient inspired leadership can thrive. They are chairpersons for the Center for Corporate Culture & Organizational Health, and founders of the International Center for Contemplative Inquiry on the Big Island of Hawaii. Their clients include NASA, World Bank, Intel, Boeing, Hewlett-Packard, Sun Microsystems, Intuit, SRI, Advanced Technologies Laboratories, and Qualcomm. West Point logisticians described their pioneering training programs for the U.S. Army Special Forces as, "the most exquisite orchestration of human technology we have ever seen." The Leveys have directed clinical mindbody programs at Group Health Cooperative of Puget Sound and at Children's Hospital in Seattle, and have served as faculty at Antioch University, Bastyr University, International Center for Organization Design, World Business Academy, and the Indian Institute of Management. They have coached several Olympic Gold and World Class record-holding athletes, as well as many CEOs and senior business leaders. The Leveys' publications include: *Living in Balance: A Dynamic Approach for Creating Harmony and Wholeness in a Chaotic World; Simple Meditation and Relaxation; Wisdom at Work;*

The Fine Art of Relaxation (CD); *The Focused Mindstate;* and *Corporate Culture and Organizational Health.* For more information on their work, programs, and publications please visit their website at www.Wisdomatwork.com

The Leveys welcome your correspondence and feedback on this book at: balance@wisdomatwork.com

▼ ▼ ▼

Wisdom Publications invites you explore in-depth some of the practices introduced in *The Fine Arts of Relaxation, Concentration, and Meditation* with these wonderful books:

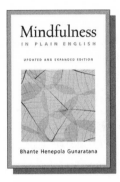

MINDFULNESS IN PLAIN ENGLISH
UPDATED AND EXPANDED EDITION
Bhante Henepola Gunaratana
224 pages, 0-86171-321-4, $14.95

With his distinctive clarity and wit, "Bhante G" teaches how meditation can truly help us live a more productive and peaceful life. This classic bestseller now includes a timely new chapter on the cultivation of compassion in a difficult world.

"Of great value to newcomers...especially people without access to a teacher."
—Larry Rosenberg, author of *Breath by Breath*

"A masterpiece. I cannot recommend it highly enough."
—Jon Kabat-Zinn, author of *Wherever You Go, There You Are*

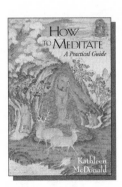

HOW TO MEDITATE
A PRACTICAL GUIDE
Kathleen McDonald
224 pages, 0-86171-009-6, $14.95

What is Tibetan Buddhist meditation? Why practice it? How do I do it? The answers to these often-asked questions are contained in this down-to-earth book written by a Western Buddhist nun with solid experience in both the practice and teaching of meditation

"This book is as beautifully simple and direct as its title." —*Yoga Today*

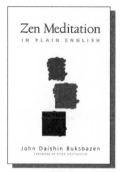

ZEN MEDITATION IN PLAIN ENGLISH

John Daishin Buksbazen ~ Foreword by Peter Matthiessen
128 pages, 0-86171-316-8, $12.95

Destined to become the classic manual for beginning instruction in Zen meditation.

"The essentials that any new practitioner needs to know to enter the Way."—John Daido Loori, abbot, Zen Mountain Monastery, editor of *The Art of Just Sitting*

"An authentic presentation of a universal and timeless teaching, particularly valuable because of the practical clarity and warmth of its style." —Dennis Gempo Merzel, Abbot of Kanzeon Zen Center, author of *Beyond Sanity and Madness*

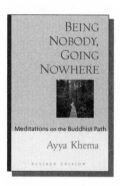

BEING NOBODY, GOING NOWHERE
MEDITATIONS ON THE BUDDHIST PATH

Ayya Khema ✦ Foreword by Zoketsu Norman Fischer
224 pages, 0-86171-198-X, $16.95

Winner of the Christmas Humphreys Award
Best Introductory Buddhist Book

In this new edition of her classic bestseller, Ayya Khema gives clear, practical instruction for overcoming counter-productive habits and beliefs.

"This jewel of a book is full of sound, practical advice. Not just highly recommended but essential reading." —*The Middle Way: Journal of the Buddhist Society*

A wealth of fine books about meditation, and Buddhism—
browse through them all at **wisdompubs.org.**

While you're there, be sure to sign up to receive the Wisdom Reader, our free monthly newsletter, for additional updates and offers.

WISDOM PUBLICATIONS

Wisdom Publications, a not-for-profit publisher, is dedicated to preserving and transmitting important works from all the major Buddhist traditions as well as related East-West themes.

To learn more about Wisdom, or browse our books on-line, visit our website at wisdompubs.org. You may request a copy of our mail-order catalog on-line or by writing to:

199 Elm Street
Somerville, Massachusetts, 02144 USA
Telephone: (617) 776-7416
Fax: (617) 536-1897

THE WISDOM TRUST

As a non-profit publisher, Wisdom is dedicated to the publication of fine Dharma books for the benefit of all sentient beings. We depend upon sponsors in order to publish books like the one you are holding in your hand.

If you would like to make a donation to the Wisdom Trust Fund to help us continue our Dharma work, or to receive information about opportunities for planned giving, please write to our Somerville office.

Thank you.

Wisdom Publications is a non-profit, charitable 501(c)(3) organization and a part of the Foundation for the Preservation of the Mahayana Tradition (FPMT).